VITALITY
A Healthy and Happy Heart

3 Keys for Sustained Weight Loss,
Type 2 Diabetes Control and Stress Management

GW00643516

Pranita Salunke
OT, MSc Preventive Cardiology

Praised by Professor David A Wood,
Emeritus Professor of Cardiology

Copyright

Powerhouse Publications
Suite 124. 94 London Road
Headington, Oxford
OX3 9FN

www.powerhousepublishing.com

Dedication

I dedicate this book:

To my mum for inspiring me to live a life of purpose.

To my dad: thank you for your unconditional love.

To my brother Tushar, for your lifelong support.

To my son Ishaan, for my reason to be.

Contents

Foreword

Pranita offers a holistic view of how to achieve the best of health, based on a wealth of experience as a health practitioner and a student of preventive cardiology at Imperial College London. She provides a clear vision of health in her book, how it can be achieved and nurtured, and offers help for everyone.

Professor David A Wood, Emeritus Professor of Cardiology, National Heart and Lung Institute, Imperial College London.

Introduction

"YOU are more powerful than your genes. The destiny of your health is determined by your lifestyle, environment, heart and mind and not only your genetic blueprint."
—Pranita Salunke

Having a truly healthy heart goes beyond being at your desired body weight and being disease-free. I believe it is also about having real joy in your heart, your ability to connect with yourself and others in a more profound and meaningful way, living a purposeful life, being truly happy from inside, and savouring life with both hands.

Science has proven that health and happiness are interconnected. Edward Diener, professor of social psychology at the University of Utah, explores subjective well-being, measuring how people evaluate their own lives, happiness, and health. According to his examinations, happy people were more likely to take better care of themselves as opposed to self-proclaimed unhappy people. Instead of resorting to an unhealthy, sedentary lifestyle, they chose healthy behaviours—like exercising, eating well, and getting adequate sleep.(1) Our sense of well-being and happiness is a precursor for helping us achieve and sustain a healthy lifestyle.

The reverse is also true – deterioration of your health may have a negative domino effect on every part of your life: finances, family, love, future goals, and notably on your levels of happiness.

Highly-driven people, business leaders, investors, entrepreneurs, people like you and me, are continually looking to optimise their health, performance, and levels of happiness because they believe in the notion that: happiness is THE basis for a successful life.

Because you are reading this book, I am sure you are one of the 'highly-driven individuals'. I encourage you to reflect on your relationship with your health and how happy and content you feel in your life at the present moment.

Ask these two important questions:

- How is my current heath level influencing my happiness in life?
- How is my level of happiness affecting my health?

Are your answers leading you to search for newer, more holistic ways to prevent chronic diseases or premature death? Is the search to optimise your health, happiness, and energy very strong in you as you realise its importance to positively influence society and create your unique legacy and savour beautiful life experiences with your loved ones? If you have answered YES, then this book will guide you in that same quest.

> ### *"Awareness is the key to personal transformation."*
> —Pranita Salunke

We begin with a self-awareness exercise that will help you to assess your holistic health and happiness level. I encourage you to complete this reflective exercise as a foundational step.

Many of my clients who have undertaken this exercise are often surprised how incredible the power of lifestyle is on every aspect of health and life. As you progress through the book and implement the ideas that are discussed here, you may enjoy an improvement in your original assessment score – including your energy level, quality and quantity of sleep, self-confidence, performance in work and life, movement, ability to effectively manage stress, emotional wellness, your intimate and other significant relationships, and much more. Overall, your life will dramatically improve when you lean into this process with trust and determination. *Vitality: A Healthy and Happy Heart* is not only about weight loss. It is about providing an insight into a holistic lifestyle to create optimum health and inner happiness. Once you master this art and skill, chronic disease management including weight loss and type 2 diabetes, are pleasant side effects. Many of my clients surprisingly told me, half-way through the programme: "I have stopped worrying about getting on the scales to weigh myself. I trust the process to give me the desired results."

In the Introduction, I share my views on how we have created the global burden of heart disease, obesity, and type 2 diabetes, and why prevention is better than cure when it comes to chronic diseases – with thought-provoking evidence.

I share my insights on how we can reverse this damage – an understanding I gained from working with hundreds of people as a clinical Occupational Therapist, Preventive Cardiology specialist, and meditation practitioner, along with my own personal learnings of overcoming depression and being overweight. I share my personal story with you to show that no matter where you are in your health journey, you can feel empowered to transform your lifestyle towards health and happiness, knowing that your essential existence is precious to humanity.

In the subsequent chapters, I share a toolkit to create:

- Emotional harmony;
- A positive mindset towards your heart health and happiness;
- Lifestyle strategies for healthy eating, sound sleep, and joyful movement;
- New lifestyle habits that become your second nature by leveraging behavioural health psychology;
- Meaning and connection in life for a peaceful, content, and successful life on your terms.

After helping many people and myself to overcome chronic health challenges with Mind-Body-Spirit principles, I feel it is my responsibility to share my insights with the world with this book.

Some of the results and stories you will get to read in the first and subsequent chapters. However, to inspire you to have a curious mind and open heart, I am sharing a case study of one of my clients, who has achieved magnificent transformation in all areas of his life, using the very same principles I share in this book.

Know that lifestyle transformation is not a once-in-a-lifetime task, it is a journey, and I wish you incredible success in walking that journey!

Pranita

Case Study

Mr Son attended my webinar which was offered via his professional association, the Chartered Institute of Management Accountants (CIMA) in June 2020.

Mr Son is a 54-year-old, typical Englishman with a long-standing accountancy practice. He is married to a supportive wife. In the past, Mr Son enjoyed an active lifestyle, including competing in national championships for fishing and winning golf tournaments. However, he had been diagnosed with rheumatoid arthritis as an 18-year-old which had gradually limited his ability to be mobile and active.

Over a 25-year period, he felt limited in his day-to-day activities and pursuing his passion of fishing and golf. He had to take about 8 paracetamols to complete one round of golf, with excruciating pain and needing a trolley to carry his bag.

He describes his long-standing situation as: "I suffer from arthritis which limits my mobility and consequently the amount of exercise I can take. I feel like I'm in a trap, I want to exercise more, but I am unable to, so I just get unhealthy – a deep downward spiral."

Mr Son could not recollect when he last had a full night's sleep, and was always awake from 2am–5am, to fall asleep until 7am. Then, he would have a heavy breakfast, regularly eating on an autopilot before dragging himself to work.

For many years, his unhealthy lifestyle was creating a huge health concern for him as he suffered from being overweight. His abdominal obesity, high blood pressure and blood sugar levels reached the pre-diabetes level.

His low energy level, combined with mental fog, forced him to take many naps and he constantly felt overwhelmed with his to-do list. He felt like he was "dragging through life."

Altogether, this lifestyle and health situation put his self-image and confidence to the level of 0 and he despised himself when looking in the mirror. In his own words, "I accepted that 'almost good' was good enough. I have accepted 'average' for the last 15 to 20 years and have stopped looking for the opportunities."

Deep down, Mr Son knew he had to do something, but didn't know the right way to do it. In the past, he had lost weight with the help of diets and personal trainers, only to stack it back once the desired target was achieved. He often felt overwhelmed with so many resources available – books, videos, weight loss clinics – and did not know the right approach for him.

He was ready to give up before he attended my webinar and heard about the holistic lifestyle transformation approach I discuss throughout this book. This was a light-bulb moment for him to decide that he was ready to try once more, ready for a bright new future!

Using a personalised bespoke approach, we worked together for 16 sessions[1] from June to October, on very similar principles that I discuss in this book. As a result, Mr Son has now completely transformed his lifestyle and has awakened the true potential that was always hidden inside him.

A few of the results achieved following this success
(Blood results changes are from July 2020–October 2020)

- Weight loss: 17 kg
- Waist reduction: Mr Son reports: "I am now 2 waist sizes smaller and I have run out of holes on the belt I have!!!!!"
- Blood sugar reduction: HbA1c: Reduced to within normal range, from 44 mmol/mol to 40 mmol/L (No more pre-diabetes)

---

[1] The duration is based on MyAction – an innovative approach to the prevention of cardiovascular disease in the community. I have integrated other holistic perspectives; the inspiration for the duration was based on this innovative approach.(2)

- C-reactive protein: 30% Reduction (from 10mg/L to 7 mg/L) [within 3 months]

We set the following objectives for his lifestyle transformation journey:

Lifestyle transformation: Education, inspiration and empowerment to achieve:

1. Lightness of being
(weight loss, aim for at least 10% weight loss in 6 months)

Mr Son went from 117 kg for more than 15 years to now below 100 kg in a matter of 3.5 months. He achieved 15% weight loss in the relatively small duration and yes, now he loves to look in the mirror and feel immense confidence.

2. Joyful and energetic movement (pain-free)

Mr Son's old life has transformed from being sedentary most days and taking 8 paracetamols to engaging in his favourite hobby of golf.

Now Mr Son really enjoys playing a full round of golf; the speed and accuracy of his shots have improved and he can carry his own clubs around the course without needing any assistance. This one measure improved his self-image and confidence to the highest level.

3. Enhanced mental clarity and focus

Mr Son now not only has physical energy, but also mental clarity and the massive drive of a 20-year-old man. Every day, he works on his newfound purpose of supporting businesspeople with his unique skills.

Other aspects of his lifestyle have also improved immensely. After the first session where we focused on mindset and connection, he sent me this feedback: "Amazingly I slept through the night on Friday and Saturday – I can't remember the last time that happened." Since then, he sleeps regularly from 9.30pm to 5.15am, waking up rejuvenated, focused and ready to positively contribute to the world. His wife is very happy that he has stopped snoring completely. (He was previously unaware that he ever did!)

He enjoys a variety of food that nourishes his mind, body and soul and never feels like he is on any 'diet'. For him, shopping consciously and preparing meals that support his new goals have become second nature – a positive lifestyle.

Because of his renewed self-worth and self-image, he is able to protect his boundaries from the negativity of certain relationships that used to pull him down; he has also strengthened the bonds in relationships that matter more – such as with his wife and good friends. He also noted that due to this entire process, he started attracting more people who are creating a positive influence in his life – including attracting more clients for his accountancy service. (This was a positive surprise!)

Emotionally, he has now gone from feeling hopeless and stressed all the time to being a great planner and executer so that he can create rather than react to his life.

He has started to enjoy life by creating a space in his life.

All these positive changes, along with the purpose exercise we did together, have now created 360-degree transformation for the direction of his life. Instead of waiting 10 to 15 years until retirement, as he did prior to the program, Mr Son now gets up at 5.15 am to work on his new business vision that will help many businesspeople to enjoy a more balanced life and be more productive.

It is safe to say that Mr Son has exceeded his goals beyond his primary objectives and expectations.

Importantly, the changes in the biomarkers happened only in a matter of 3 to 4 months.

However, Mr Son has a strong motivation to continuously evolve into a better version of himself with this Mind-Body-Spirit integration process; 6 to 12 months in the future he will be enjoy a feeling of eternal youthfulness, optimum health and inner happiness that cannot be measured by numbers but can only be felt in his soul.

Dear readers above success is a possibility for you as well, and this is my wish for you,

Pranita

Disclaimer

The tools we discuss throughout the book are intended for people with chronic diseases and those who are looking to optimise their existing levels of health and happiness. If you are suffering with genetic conditions including type 1 diabetes, please use this information as an adjunct to your current medical treatment.

If your chronic conditions are uncontrolled, these tools must be used in addition to your medical treatment with the support of your health care provider.

Self-Awareness Exercise
Vitality: Self-Assessment

This Vitality Self-Assessment tool aims at helping you to become more self-aware of your well-being. The experience is like holding a mirror in front of you: showing your positives and aspects you could improve in.

On the scale of 0–10, how much you can relate with these statements?

0: Untrue.
10: Very true.

1. My energy levels help me to be productive at work and enjoy my life to the fullest.

2. My immediate family members haven't suffered from type 2 diabetes or early heart disease or stroke or any other chronic diseases

3. I am satisfied with my health and have stable[2] health markers such as:

    - Blood pressure
    - Blood glucose
    - Cholesterol
    - Heart age
    - Any other chronic condition.

4. I am concerned about the possibility of my health affecting my performance at work and in life.

    If yes, what are your concerns precisely?

5. I am aware of the food and lifestyle choices I have to make to maintain the highest health, energy, and well-being.

---

[2] Please contact your health professional if you are unaware of your health markers.

6. I have a healthy digestion and am able to enjoy healthy food with my loved ones.

7. I enjoy peaceful and uninterrupted sleep at night.

8. I have supple and pain-free joints and a body that helps me to be active in my hobbies and fitness of my choice.

9. I can quickly assess signs of stress and use various meditation and mind tools to manage stress effectively.

10. I experience peace, joy, and happiness on the majority of days. These feelings permeate into all critical aspects of my life and business.

11. I am at peace within myself (emotionally content) and know that I live a life filled with passion and have a purposeful occupation aligned with my values and beliefs.

12. I have a strong connection with my loved ones, my co-workers, and notably with myself.

13. Now you are aware of your health and happiness levels, what one thing you would like to change/improve?

    Use this space to write health and wellness vision and goals you wish to achieve.

    -
    -
    -

14. I am highly motivated to make positive lifestyle changes now.

CHAPTER 1

The Big Picture

An unhealthy lifestyle and stress trigger the development of Cardiovascular Diseases (CVD), their risk factors, and even certain forms of cancer. Therefore, these lifestyle-influenced diseases are strongly preventable. However, unfortunately, the rate of these lifestyle-influenced diseases is continually rising.

CVDs are caused when there is narrowing and hardening of the blood vessels of our vital organs. This manifests in various forms, such as heart attack, stroke, peripheral arterial disease, and vascular dementia.(1)

CVDs are the leading cause of death worldwide, taking an estimated 17.9 million lives each year, accounting for 31% of all deaths globally.(2) The rate is projected to increase by 50% in 2030.(3)

Even in the United Kingdom (UK), CVDs are a significant cause of death and disability; in 2011 alone, they contributed to 30% of the country's death rate.(1)

Eighty per cent of CVD deaths occur in low- and middle-income countries, creating devastating financial implications on their already-stretched economies.(2)

CVDs have severe economic implications: in 2010/2011, it cost the UK's National Health Service (NHS) £7.72 billion out of its £107 billion annual budget.(3) Harvard School of Public Health warns us against the global financial burden of these conditions. The total global cost of CVDs is set to rise from approximately US$863 billion in 2010 to a staggering US$1,044 billion by 2030.(4)

The rate of childhood obesity and type 2 diabetes has increased globally. According to the World Health Organisation, over 41 million children were overweight or obese in 2016, creating a lifetime risk of diabetes, heart disease, and a host of other metabolic conditions.(5) On the one hand, people feed themselves excessively – creating complications of obesity and CVDs, which are killing people every minute. On the other hand, young children and adults are dying from hunger and malnourishment across the world.

According to UNICEF, hunger and undernutrition contribute to more than half of global child deaths, taking the lives of approximately 3.1 million children each year. Malnourishment makes our future generations more vulnerable to illness and diseases.(6)

What are we as a society doing wrong? Unless concrete actions are taken to prevent and effectively manage the CVDs, their steady rise and risk will continue to take more lives each year.(1,3)

Quality of Life (QOL)

Even those who are lucky to survive from these conditions' complications may experience deterioration in their quality of life (QOL), as they suffer from symptoms of the conditions or side effects of heavy pharmaceutical management.

It is a struggle to manage medications and their side-effects. Dealing with the residual effects of chronic disease is a daily struggle that includes: fatigue; sleep apnoea; joint pain from carrying excess weight; symptoms of uncontrolled diabetes; and frequent trips to the bathroom which affects the quality of your sleep.

These symptoms could create a host of other conditions such as depression, diminished sex life (blood supply to the intimate part is also compromised), hospitalisation due to complications, reduced work performance, productivity loss, and this list goes on.

At a family level, compromised QOL leads to relationship strain. We can't optimally fulfil our duties towards our parents, spouse, or kids, and our communications are confounded, with the emotional stress of the symptoms.

There are profound financial implications at a family level due to the cost of medications, surgery, and time off to recuperate after any complications. At an extreme, the cost of losing a productive family member places a substantial financial strain and emotional loss. It creates a domino-distress effect on other family members.

Along with compromised quality and quantity of life, people who have heart disease, diabetes, and are overweight are at a significant risk of getting infected by severe infections. The global pandemic of COVID-19 has proven the scale of this problem with a grave significance. The government body, the UK and European Centre for Disease Prevention and Control (ECDC), informs us that uncontrolled chronic diseases, including obesity and diabetes, make us more susceptible to getting a serious infection, including COVID-19.(7)

Given the significant scale of these lifestyle conditions, wouldn't you agree that, *unless we take a proactive preventive approach for this global tsunami of CVDs, they have the power to destroy mankind?*

I believe that with the human and financial losses and the profound impact of lifestyle-influenced diseases, an effective prevention strategy must be a global priority and all individuals' responsibility.

Now that you may be motivated to focus on the prevention and reversal of these chronic conditions, let's briefly understand what factors increase the risk of developing them in the first place.

Heredity

Many people don't realise that the role of heredity in the development of CVDs and their risk factors is much smaller than other causes. There are specific genes transmitted by heredity that increase the risk of a family history of chronic conditions, including obesity, type 2 diabetes, and heart disease, making you more predisposed to developing them yourself.

For example, a gene called the fat mass and obesity-associated gene (FTO) makes it difficult for the person to limit their caloric intake.

The gene, present in up to 43% of the population, controls their eating behaviour by increasing hunger levels, reducing satiety, and increasing the tendency to be sedentary and store body fat.(8)

People from a specific ethnicity are likely to have certain conditions. For example, those of Asian, East Indian, Native American, Pacific Island, or Middle Eastern descent have a higher risk of being insulin resistant, setting the stage for obesity or being overweight.(9)

Yet, even if you are carrying these 'defective genes,' you must not feel powerless.

> *'You are only predisposed, not pre-destined for developing lifestyle-related conditions.*
> *Transforming your lifestyle, you can positively influence your gene expression.'*
> —Pranita Salunke

Evidence from epigenetics[3] and twin studies suggests that our thoughts, environment, and lifestyle behaviour can influence which of our genes are turned on or off.(10) In other words, even if you are carrying specific genes from your ancestors, if you choose a positive lifestyle, there are higher chances that you will remain healthy.

The role of environment and lifestyle choices is so powerful that an American physician and *New York Times* best-selling author Dr Mark Hyman states very boldly (11):

> "Genetics loads the gun, but environment pulls the trigger."

---

[3] Epigenetics: The study of organisms' changes caused by modification of gene expression rather than alteration of the genetic code itself.

Along with genetics, our environment and lifestyle choices and their interactions influence the risk of acquiring a chronic disease [G×E].(12)

I am sharing this information with you to EMPOWER you. You can take control of your health destiny by transforming your lifestyle, positively influencing your environment, and reducing the incidences of chronic disease significantly – both as an individual and collectively as a society.

"YOU are more powerful than your GENES!"
—Pranita Salunke

Lifestyle-related (Preventable) causes of CVDs:

A growing body of scientific research suggests that chronic disease risks are strongly lifestyle-related and preventable.

"80% of premature heart disease,
stroke and diabetes can be prevented."
—World Health Organisation (13)

I would invite you to look at the table below and examine which of these lifestyle risk factors relate to you – then transform your lifestyle, and replace with proactive, preventive measures to the best of your abilities.(14)

Preventable CVD risk factors and unhealthy lifestyle habits:
- Tobacco use,
- Poor diet of refined, ready-made and processed food,
- Physical inactivity,
- The harmful use of alcohol,
- Being overweight,
- Abdominal obesity (more fat around your visceral organs is particularly detrimental to your heart health,
- Diabetes,
- High blood pressure.

Heart Age score:

NHS, UK, has produced a tool that gives you your heart age compared to your real age.(15) As an awareness exercise, I would recommend you take this test to keep you motivated to act on heart health. You can find it here: https://www.nhs.uk/conditions/nhs-health-check/check-your-heart-age-tool/

Before moving on to behaviour changes that you need to adapt, it will be valuable to understand how we have reached this global burden of lifestyle-related diseases, lesser known to our ancestors who enjoyed long, healthy, and happy lives.

Why are we as a society experiencing the negative impact of these lifestyle-related diseases, even with advancements in healthcare, diet and nutritional guidelines, and easy accessibility to physical activity centres and services available to stop smoking or alcohol habits?

Is reversing CVD's risk with weight loss and disease control merely a function of calories in and calories out and taking therapeutic drugs?

I think there is more to living a healthy life than our narrow focus on these measures.

Society's role in creating lifestyle disease

Our ancestors enjoyed cooking and eating food close to nature, and being physically active throughout the day in meaningful occupations such as working on farms and growing their own food, sharing love, and being closely connected with family and their community.

Modern man has made remarkable progress in science, technology, and innovation. But there are some severe side effects to this advancement. There is an advancement in the way we eat our food from genetically-modified seeds to food that travels thousands of air miles and the vast majority of chemicals used to preserve the food on our shelves. In the current fast-paced world, there is enormous pressure on meeting time-work-personal demands. Therefore food, diet, and pharmaceutical industries are investing millions of pounds to make people's lives 'easier' – or so they say.

Every day, we hear of a new product launch, giving us a variety of tempting options – pleasure-producing, convenient, processed, and preserved food packaged attractively and marketed at the grass-roots level across the globe.

We are relying on packaged food from a very young age – from drinking formula milk to first fruit purees, quenching our thirst with soda and sugary juices, to quickly getting off-the-shelf sandwiches and prepared food ready to be heated and consumed sitting in front of our screens. As a result of eating a packaged, processed, ready-made 'western diet' for decades, it is no wonder that a variety of lifestyle illnesses are on the rise.

With an allure of modernisation, this ready-made lifestyle is now adopted in Eastern and more traditional cultures, including South Asia, South America, and some Mediterranean countries.

To control these illnesses, pharmaceutical companies are ready with newer drug approaches that may give a temporary symptomatic relief rather than addressing the root cause.

To add to this confusion, different experts promote different diet styles. For example, one expert praises a low-calorie diet while another recommends a low-carb diet, and yet another a high protein -low-fat diet.

The changing work culture has forced us to sit for long hours at a desk, unlike our ancestors who moved throughout their day working on the farm or in the community.

In the past, we lived with extended families or in a community. However, migration in search of a better life has fragmented the extended family and created more nuclear families worldwide. As a result, challenges of social isolation, disconnection, and lack of community support are on the rise.

I have personally experienced the dire effects of social isolation, which led me to depression. When I relocated from India to the UK in 2005, a lack of community support and other physical challenges (such as the extremes of weather and the different culture), shocked my physiology and mental health. It affected all areas of my life, including health, career success, and relationships.

The shift to a nuclear-family society has created an influx of psychological distress of varying degrees, from general discomfort to lack of self-care motivation. People are fearful of reaching out to new people – they would much rather sit in the comfort of their home, eating dinner in front of the TV, or communicating via email or text. Can you relate to this situation?

This environment creates a downward spiral of excessive drinking, seeking foods, drinks, and drugs to fill that emotional void, indulging in poor lifestyle habits, and relying on medicines and surgery to compensate for chronic disease complications.

Work and life stress – such as lack of control over work and marital conflicts – lead to risky behaviours such as smoking, excessive drinking, and sedentary behaviours.(15) Various guidelines use these behaviours as indicators to predict the risk of developing heart diseases.(14)

Admittedly, medical or surgical interventions become necessary once chronic lifestyle-related diseases are already established and are creating their complications.

However, my professional experience and observation is that, triggering an 'unhealthy lifestyle' is the emotional distress and mind-body disconnection the person is experiencing.

These lifestyle habits and behaviours are created and instilled by deep-seated influences such as the environment, values passed on by social culture, family and friends, as well as lack of meaningful and purposeful occupation.

What is the ROOT problem?

Mind: Chronic life stresses lead to feelings of depression, anxiety, stress, and social isolation.

Body: Unhealthy eating, lack of quality and quantity of sleep, sedentary lifestyle.

Connection: Absence of meaningful and purposeful work and weak relationship with self and others.

When we focus on mere willpower to make changes to diet, physical activities, or sleep, they are short-term, giving us temporary results. Hence, to create a sustainable Lifestyle Transformation that prevents chronic diseases and helps us to savour life to the fullest, we have to work on the approach that acts on the three levels of Mind, Body, and Connection.

I present *Vitality: the mind-body-connection principles*:

- Strengthening connections with ourselves and our community; living a life of passion and purpose.
- Creating a healthy mindset and shifting negative emotions into positive ones.
- Adopting and sustaining healthy lifestyle behaviours of savouring healthy food, moving joyfully, and enjoying restful sleep.

The pleasant result for you if you embrace this approach will be:

- Achieving your ideal weight,
- Control of chronic diseases including type 2 diabetes or high blood pressure.
- Enjoying peace, calm, clarity, and happiness.
- Infusing yourself with vital energy and enthusiasm.
- Ultimately, you achieve a healthy and happy heart that beats stronger for longer.

I believe both the quantity and quality of our lives can be improved if we approach our heart health from inside out.

My story

The aforementioned statistics are not just printed numbers. There are real people like you and me behind those figures.

I had to learn this the hard way. In 2007, both my maternal uncle and my first cousin left the world in their 40s, leaving behind families, due to type 2 diabetes complications – a very real loss behind the statistics.

Both of my losses could have been preventable with lifestyle transformation. I felt frustrated as I couldn't do anything at the time – even with my clinical experience; even when I was aware of the science behind these conditions.

At the same time, I worked in the NHS as an occupational therapist, witnessing people coming in for different treatments: amputation, heart surgery, liver, kidney failures, and living a poor quality of life and dying early. The precursor of these endpoints were chronic lifestyle-related conditions such as obesity and diabetes. I felt frustrated both professionally and personally.

That's when I started pursuing my advanced Preventive Cardiology training at Imperial College London. This experience gave me a fresher perspective on how I could create positive changes in the way I served my clients.

Eminent Professor David Wood, our course director, was my inspiration to start this wellness service. He authored national and international guidelines on the Prevention of Cardiovascular Diseases and was very scientific in his approach, yet he encouraged my practice of mindfulness and meditation. I am immensely grateful for that encouragement, which helped me regain my confidence. This empowered me to create a wellness program that uses my existing skills of Occupational Therapist (counselling for healthy behaviour changes) and integrates into evidence-based Preventive Cardiology advice on all aspects of lifestyle to achieve a healthy heart and control lifestyle diseases.

In my approach, I also include my passion and life-long learnings of yoga and meditation practices because they have helped my clients and me enormously in achieving a sense of wellness.

I call this the Vitality Mind-Body-Connection (MBC) approach, as it not only assists people to control chronic diseases but also infuses them with optimum health, energy, clarity, and inner joy.

I felt like I had found my purpose: to inspire people to embrace a positive lifestyle to enjoy a healthy heart, lead a purposeful life, and share happiness with their loved ones.

As the Vitality MBC approach started giving positive results for my clients, I felt excited and enthusiastic to continue my journey. Now, I had the knowledge and confidence to bring about the change, one person and one health behaviour at a time.

With this book, I wish to enthusiastically share this integrative approach with the intention that, even if one person gets inspired by this message and it prevents their health complications, one precious life is saved, and I will fulfil my purpose.

You have taken an essential first step by opening this book. As you find joy in the meditations, lifestyle and psychological tools described here, you will ready yourself to step into your highest self, your dream health and body, sharp and focused mind and loving heart, that spread joy to yourself and others.

Vitality: A Healthy and Happy Heart is a complete guide for preparing yourself to live life to the fullest. Let us start the journey together towards your healthy and happy heart!

Positive results using Vitality-Mind-Body Connection principles to inspire you! (*..Names are changed)

- Dear Pranita, It is quite hard to put into words my gratitude and thanks for all your help and advice that you have given me over the last few months. As you know, I am your best customer: I have type two diabetes and have had a heart attack and a double heart bypass five and six years ago respectively. I made the decision back in February that I wanted to change my lifestyle. I was fed up with being a yo-yo dieter and that meant that my sugar levels were too high and that leads to all sorts of health issues and problems. I think you would admit that I was quite a difficult person to get into the plan initially. I have an extremely busy lifestyle with two teenage daughters and my business; I found it quite difficult to adapt to the change in lifestyle. There was so much to remember and do (or not) with what, when, and how much I was eating as well as controlling stress levels. I'm sure you remember that I quit the program in the past several times – but you were there for me being very positive, and encouraging me to continue. Now, after four months, I can sincerely say that you have changed my life. I'm extremely positive about my future health. The aim was to lose some weight and I have gone from just over 15 stones to just under 15 stones – so 8 pounds. That may not sound like a rapid weight loss, but the key for me is to do the changes I have made slowly so they become a habit and permanent. Most importantly, I went to see my diabetic specialist on Tuesday. Now, I have not seen him for a year and his first words to me were: "You look well." My sugar levels have now dropped from a dangerously-high level six months ago to below the diabetic threshold. My specialist told me effectively that I do not have diabetes anymore! I'm really focused now on getting my levels and weight down even further and this is all down to you. You have given me the education and tools to not only consider what and how much I'm eating, but you have also worked on the mental and visualization side of it as well. Your motto, "What goes in your head is as important as what goes in your mouth" is so true. Thank you for everything you have done for me. I am so grateful. – Mr Smith.

- "I have lost over a stone in weight. However, even more remarkably, my recent blood test shows that I'm no longer pre-diabetic. My cholesterol levels have come down 27%, and my heart age has improved by 14 years. I also have more energy than I've had for many years." – Mr R.

- "People say I look much younger and healthier than 18 months ago, and I lost 22 kg." – Mr Ross.

- "I would like to thank Pranita for the excellent delivery of the Vitality health programme which both my wife and I enrolled on. Pranita is a very knowledgeable and experienced individual who is passionate about what she does. My biggest issue was getting a good night's sleep and she worked with me to address this. She started by analysing the medical reports and blood tests and then tailored her advice. She was able to give some very useful practical tips on various health-related matters and also advised us on healthy food choices. I would definitely recommend Pranita to others seeking a helping hand in looking after their health and wellbeing. Thank you." – Mr Patel.

- "I just wanted to express my thanks to Pranita for arranging the Vitality Health Programme. It was an excellent course on how to make the most of one's health and live with vitality. Pranita, you are doing a great job in the wellness and health industry; I believe this programme will change people's lives into being the healthiest and happiest. God bless you!!!" – Mr Tuscano.

- "Pranita Salunke is not only highly experienced and knowledgeable, she goes the extra mile to diagnose and understand her clients by building strong rapport. She has very good practical tips on managing stress and improving wellbeing. I would definitely recommend her and the positive energy she brings." – Mr Smith.

- "I've been a yo-yo dieter for over 30 years. At my highest weight last summer (2015), I had an enormous wardrobe of clothes that didn't fit me. I was uncomfortable in the heat and suffered from puffy ankles/lower legs. Worst of all, I had developed an anxiety around my weight and general health. I began working with Pranita because I knew I had to break the yo-yo dieting cycle and take a different approach in order to feel and become healthier, lose weight – and keep it off. When I first met with Pranita, the main thing that struck me was how non-judgmental she was – and how positive. She encouraged me to look not backwards to past failures, but positively towards future success. She began the work of shifting my mindset from diet to healthy lifestyle very gently, whilst never losing focus on the essential need to lose weight. She introduced me to some of her core philosophies, whilst making me feel excited about her approach and the help she could give me. Pranita used coaching and NLP techniques and encouraged me to work with visualisations and affirmations to great effect, especially in incorporating regular exercise into my lifestyle. Her advice on healthy food choices has been helpful too. With Pranita's support, I've been able to eliminate almost all added/refined sugar and simple carbohydrates from my diet – something I'm immensely grateful to have achieved. The eight sessions ran across six months and I lost over three stone (44 pounds/20 kilo). I'm delighted with this result and am continuing with the healthy habits I've adopted, with the aim of losing more weight. With Pranita's support I dropped more than 3 dress sizes and I'm wearing clothes that haven't fitted me for over 10 years. Most notable of all is that the anxieties I'd been feeling over my state of health have receded significantly. I would recommend

Pranita for these reasons: 1. There is an integrity in this process and in Pranita, which is very reassuring. There is nothing 'faddy' or short-term about Pranita's programme – it is fit for life, very sustainable 'best practice'. 2. The combination of focus on (i) eating/healthy food choices, (ii) exercise/activity, and (iii) mental/psychological support is excellently balanced and invaluable – a truly holistic approach. 3. I really appreciated the way Pranita helps her clients embed new healthier habits one by one, and does not try to make them change everything at once. It feels a less radical and much more manageable way to achieve a lasting transformation. 4. There's a real value in being supported through a few weeks or better still, a few months of habit-change. Making the changes to a healthier lifestyle doesn't happen overnight, and it's too easy to give up when the struggle gets too much. With the ongoing support through Pranita's programme, it is possible not only to adopt new habits, but to make them stick. – Ms Shela.

• I very much enjoyed attending a "Care Workshop" given by Pranita. Her approach is both engaging and persuasive. Pranita speaks with great passion on topics related to an all-round healthy lifestyle. She's clearly knowledgeable on the mental, physical and emotional aspects, as well as being understanding of the foibles of the human condition – which means that most of us tend to know what we should do to stay healthy, yet still struggle to do it. The workshop gave her audience a taster of Pranita's professional approach to motivating, informing and supporting her clients to achieve their health and wellbeing goals – and passed on some practical mental and physical exercises too. Having seen Pranita address a room full of businesspeople with essentially sedentary jobs, one can be in no doubt of the extent of her understanding and empathy – and her desire to make a difference. – Mr Hoffman.

- I have always believed in a healthy lifestyle, but for the past few years I have let work and life get in the way of what was important. When I read the information about your 6-week Vitality Energiser Course, I knew it was the right decision for Lydia and I to get started on a journey to health. Working in a small group we learnt the right way to eat, to exercise and to enjoy life but more than that, we understood why. You showed us that being healthy doesn't have to be boring or painful, and it's not about numbers on a scale. With small adjustments to our diet and the right tips for exercise, Lydia and I have improved our lives in ways that we couldn't even imagine. The goals that we set for ourselves are close to being achieved. I have yet to try a length underwater, but with my improved stamina I will very soon. The reason I am writing this is not just because of the quality of the course, but the way you made yourself available to us outside of it, motivating us, inspiring us and guiding us, not just as individuals but as a group, organising social gatherings and keeping us on our journey. You give yourself wholeheartedly, truly believing in what you do. Your passion is only matched by your compassion, positivity and energy. I know that Lydia and I will be coming back to you to continue our journey in the future and I have and will continue to recommend your amazing services to friends, relatives and colleagues. – Mr Goldsmith.

- "I'd like to thank you for the help and support you gave me in our last Vitality Health Clinic session. As you well know, I've long been suffering from complex health problems – problems that when managed by a disciplined diet, healthy lifestyle and the right kind of thinking can be significantly reduced. A session with you was the catalyst to changes that I have now begun making in my lifestyle. I am happy to report I'm now beginning to see the beneficial effects. Most impressive was the unexpected impact you had on my thought processes and perspective, and you achieved this from just some simple questioning and relaxation exercises. I'll happily and confidently recommend you to others in the future. With sincere thanks." – Nick Rhodes.

- "I just wanted to express my thanks to you for your Vitality Health Programme. It was an excellent course on how to make the most of one's health and live with vitality. Generally, we think being healthy is just about food and exercise, i.e. less calories in and more exercise results in weight loss = good health. Thanks for busting that myth! I was amazed at the different aspects you worked on with us: head-space/mindset/breathing/visualisations/resolution setting when in a heightened physiological state/high alkaline body state/getting your gut flora back/super foods. I've found the course motivational, allowing me to identify what I was doing well and what I need to work on. I would highly recommend it to anyone who wants to have a healthy and happy future. Thank you again!" – Ms Jackson.

- "I just wanted to say a huge thank you. Before I came to see you, I was worried about my weight and health. Added to this, my blood tests showed I was pre-diabetic and a number of my blood levels were at an unhealthy level. You created a personal programme for me that addressed my specific health and weight loss issues. In our weekly check-ups, you monitored my progress and advised me when and how I should make changes to ensure I was on track and gave me constant encouragement, support and motivation. After just five weeks I have lost over a stone in weight. However, even more remarkably, my recent blood tests show that I'm no longer pre-diabetic, my cholesterol levels have come down 27% and my heart age has improved by 14 years. In addition, I have more energy than I've had for many years. Most importantly, you've shown me how to make the changes to more nutritional food and exercise that are now part of my normal weekly routine, so I'm confident I can maintain this as a permanent part of my healthier lifestyle. I'm so grateful for all the care, attention and expert advice you've given me and the results you've helped me to achieve in such a short period of time. Thank you once again." – Mr Howards.

SECTION 1

Connection: With Yourself

"Nurture your ultimate life vision by achieving optimum health and inner happiness."
—Pranita Salunke

CHAPTER 2

Inspiration, Intention and Visualisation

I believe inspiration is a strong force that pulls you towards adopting and sustaining a positive lifestyle. The force is even stronger than motivation. Motivation may last as long as you have strong willpower. However, when life's other responsibilities dominate, many people fail to sustain that willpower, and hence any changes they have adopted are short-lived.

The following statistics are a clear evidence for this (1):

- 87% of people who try to quit smoking fail within one year.
- 81% of people who go on a diet fail to stick with it after one year.
- 92% of people who set New Year's resolutions fail at their attempt.

(The University of Scranton found only 8 % of people who make resolutions meet their goal. Psychologists have named this 'false hope syndrome'.)

If you want to be among those select few who make their vision of optimum health and vitality by transforming their lifestyle and mindset, you have to be in the state of INSPIRATION.

When you are inspired, you live "in spirit", says successful author and motivational speaker Dr Wayne Dyer.(2) When your actions and lifestyle choices are aligned with your SPIRIT, you are powerful.

The Power of Intention

Inspiration is directly related to the strength of your intention to achieve your health goals.

A pioneer of integrative medicine, Dr Deepak Chopra, affirms that intention has a creative power. When you set the intention to achieve your deepest desires by being calm and centred (like you are in a meditative state), then you will observe universal forces orchestrating in symphony to fulfil your deepest desires. So, let us use this knowledge and visualise your ultimate life vision supported by optimum health and wellness.

"Intention has infinite organising power."
– Deepak Chopra, *The Spontaneous Fulfilment of Desire*

Visualisation exercise:

During this visualisation meditation, you may get intuition, an idea, an aha moment that will assist you in achieving your health vision, so I encourage you to keep a notebook and pen next to you, (You can also listen to this video I have created: https://pranitavitality.com/video/).

1. Sit in a quiet place with soothing lights, wearing comfortable clothes, away from distraction and noise either in a chair or on a mat on the floor, wherever you feel comfortable.

   Now, with eyes closed, relax your body and bring your attention to your breathing. As you observe your breathing, you will notice it will slow down automatically. Keep following your breathing; if your mind wanders for a few moments, observe it, and then slowly bring it back to your breathing.

2. Gradually, you will notice your thoughts are fading away like clouds passing over a clear blue sky. You will clear your consciousness of thoughts and move into a positive state of being. You will experience a state of restful awareness.

3. Usually, our mind is occupied with different thoughts and feelings from the past or concerns of the future, making it difficult to connect with our highest self and the present moment where our real power lies. But right now, you are entering a creative space of pure consciousness.

4. Smile with your whole body as deep long inhalations fill you up with positive energy, and return to the world on exhalation.

5. Imagine warm orange energy of pure sunlight circulating from the top of your head to your chest, to your stomach. The energy is warming up your legs, going down deep into the earth, circulating back to the top of your head.

6. With every inhale-exhale, you are glowing brighter and brighter. You are now becoming one with that orange light.

7. Feel it with all your senses. See the colours swirling around your face, your whole body like the powerful sun.

8. You have the power of the sun.

9. If you are that powerful, what can you achieve? Anything you desire!

10. Now is the time to ask the question: what are my life desires? What do I really want?

Visualise your intentions of a slender, energised body, healthy blood levels, and healthy heart, increasing happiness in your life becoming your reality.

- What will it mean to you? How will your loved ones benefit? What will you achieve?
- How it will enhance your own and your loved ones' happiness?
- How it will strengthen other areas of your life?
- How will the success of this one goal contribute to your life's vision?
- How will you feel after you are successful at being healthy and happy?
- With enhanced energy, enthusiasm, and passion, you are now able to lead a purposeful and impactful life, and significantly contribute to society by leaving your unique legacy.

You may visualise:

"I feel proud of myself for making positive changes, and it is so easy, to travel, go to meetings, to the places without worrying about managing medications. I feel happy that I am a good role model for my kids. I feel confident to look into the mirror. The positive lifestyle I am making has resulted in a fabulous physique, which makes me feel proud.

With this increased confidence, I am more likely to pursue my promotion/new job/that dream career or business to enhance my financial well-being.

I can go on trips I resisted in the past due to health conditions.

I feel Free.
I feel Powerful.
I Feel Safe.
I feel Happy!"

Affirm to yourself:

"I am healthy, happy, and energetic.
I am powerful beyond my wildest dreams.
I am a beautiful soul inside and out.
I love and appreciate the functioning of my body's cells, my mind's creativity, and my compassionate heart."

Enjoy this blissful creative process for few more minutes before becoming aware of your breathing again – breathe in and breathe out. Gradually become aware of your environment and open your eyes.

- As you progress, throughout your day, carry the warm orange light and power of the sun you experienced in the meditation to bring you more energy, vitality, clarity, confidence, love, peace, and joy.
- Namaste.

A note: Do not get attached to the outcome or worry about when you will achieve success. TRUST that your intentions are now released in the pure potential of the expansive universe. If you hold on to this vision and take positive, inspired actions, you will soon lead a path to optimum health and happiness.

Leverage The Pain

While many people are often pulled towards the glorious vision of their health, occasionally, some are also inspired to action by thinking of the pain associated with staying at their current health level. If this is you, consider reflecting on the following questions about your goals:

- What will it cost me to stay at this same level of health and wellness?
- What has it cost me in the past?
- How are the people I love affected by my current health status?
- How is my (—work, family, business) being affected by my health?

The important question is **whether to make changes or remain the same** NOW?

Both of the above exercises will bring positive and negative emotions; both will help you find your WHY: your reasons to create positive changes.

My firm belief is that if you find strong reasons to accomplish your goals and, importantly, get connected with those reasons regularly, a sustained inspiration will be ensured on the days you feel like giving up. When an external situation demands that you give up on your positive lifestyle – for example, the weather outside is terrible, or when you have a conflict at work – your strong reasons will keep you inspired to act.

Vision Board:

You have tuned into your success feelings and found your WHY to succeed in your goals. Now capture these emotions on a vision board. The board will act as a visual cue and an inspiration to work daily to attain your dreams. In his famous book, *Think and Grow Rich*, author Napoleon Hill, emphasises the importance of visualising the accomplishment of your goals, morning and night. When you envision, you are already living a positive future in the current moment.

Remember the emotions you experienced during the visualisation process when you saw yourself shining with optimum health and vitality? Now, search for images that evoke those emotions.

You could stick these images on a board, or you can also create a computer version of the vision board, but I encourage a physical one, which appears more real to your senses, and is therefore more powerful.

Importantly, look at your vision board, day and night. You may have put an image of a healthy, energetic, well-dressed, affluent man or woman confidently doing business deals. Or you may be cruising across the ocean, living your adventures like travelling, skydiving, running a marathon, or enjoying your favourite sports of golf and tennis. You may be in your beloved's arms, with newfound self-love, confidence and health; you may have attracted your perfect partner with ease.

Close your eyes and put yourself in the same space as in the image. I recommend playing lively music in the background, and using all your senses: looking at the surroundings you are in and what food you are tasting. How loved do you feel? Can you feel the breeze of the ocean on your skin?

Savour your vision with all your senses.

CHAPTER 3

Empowering Beliefs For Optimum Health

"When our mind-body-spirit is connected, we are happy,
healthy, and whole."
—Pranita Salunke

Power of beliefs

Just like a spider's web, our mind is made up of a beautiful intricate design. Threads we gather throughout our lives – our childhood environment, positive or negative experiences from our friends, parents and teachers – ensure the strength or weakness of that structure upon which we build our lives.

If the structure is strong, we THRIVE, but its weakness halts our progress in all areas of our life: health, wealth, and meaningful relationships. To truly savour life, we need to feel successful in all these three dimensions – do you agree?

What is the point of being just materially successful if you have to pop pills to keep your heart pumping or drink copious amounts of caffeine to stay awake to work on your business way past midnight? These actions would drain your energy, and you would have nothing left for yourself, your passions, and your relationships.

Ask yourself:

If you didn't have any limitations in your mind, where would your dreams and desire take you in your life?

What new mind-threads do you need to create to erase the old and build the new YOU?

Set the intention to break the obstacles that present themselves as mental bindings limiting your ability to achieve your health goals.

Just like the success of my dear client Mr Robson who struggled to achieve the ideal weight for many years, you will be able to create a new mental foundation upon which you can build a beautiful structure for your health. Mr Robson tried many different diets, restricting calories, going to weight loss support groups (like Weight Watchers); he would lose some weight and regain after a few months. His gradually increasing weight was concerning to him as his blood test was showing signs of metabolic conditions. He started feeling despair and hopelessness. But the inner voice inside him kept him searching for the ideal way to reach his healthy weight and he was determined to make a positive shift in his health. He found inspiration in his desire to fit into a three-sizes-smaller suit to wear at his wedding, set in a French chalet overlooking the ocean in 8 months' time. Together, we used the power of meditation to enhance his self-worth, confidence, and the possibility of achieving his optimum health. As a result, he was able to sustain positive changes of sound sleep, better movement, strengthening relationships, and savouring healthy food. After 8 months, he joyfully took a flight to southern France in the summer, where he showed off his newfound confidence – three and a half stones lighter and healthier in his beautiful off-white suit. All his relatives couldn't believe his transformation, but he knew that it was due to the change in his level of consciousness and mindset.

Mr Robson's story echoes what many of us have felt at some point in our lives. After a few (or many) unsuccessful attempts at weight loss with different diets and exercise programs, it's easy to give up and stop believing that we have control over our health destiny or that the right approach suited to our unique needs exists.

Inner Conflict

We have a deep desire to look and feel at our best, feel healthy and energetic throughout the day, and positively impact our presence. Our heart wants that, but our mind insists it's not possible, and we experience inner conflict with ourselves.

One part of our self is screaming, "Yes, I deserve to be at my ideal weight, healthy and energetic!" While another part insists, "What's the point? I tried so many times, and still, my health situation is the same." When there is a tug-of-war between our beliefs and desires, the stress it creates paralyses and prevents us from recognising our innate worth for achieving the optimum health that is our birthright.

Our beliefs create the experiences we have in our lives, both positives, and negatives. If you believe, "I am in the process of finding the right plan to achieve my ideal weight and it is easy to make those changes," then that will be your experience. On the other hand, if your belief is that type 2 diabetes (or any other lifestyle-related diseases) are in our family, so "What's the use of choosing a healthy lifestyle or trying to be healthy? I am destined for the disease!" then eventually that will become your reality. Respecting some heredity risk elements, as we discussed in the first chapter, WE have more control over our health.

So, believing and trusting that you deserve to enjoy optimum health, a slender body, and high energy is an essential first step in achieving your desired health success.

To build and strengthen your belief, start looking for evidence that it is a possibility for you. Read as many success stories as Mr Robson in your network, community, or on the Internet. The point is to keep believing that if other people can successfully overcome their weight and health struggles, then so can you. Nurture the belief that, "My ideal health exists, and I am in the process of discovering the route to it."

Break through the negative beliefs

You also have to break through the negative beliefs that you may have been living with since childhood. For example, do you believe that achieving optimum health and weight is even a possibility for you? If you struggled for many years, you might doubt yourself, but let me tell you that one part of you still believes in its possibility; otherwise, you may have stopped your search and not read this book.

Consider if you resonate with some of these common beliefs that create limitations in our health success:

- I have always been a big person.
- I love my food, and weight loss means giving up my joy; I want to enjoy my life.
- How I look doesn't matter, what matters is my money in the bank and my work ethics.
- I have tried many times; what's the point in exploring a new approach? It will be all the same.
- I am too old to change.
- I don't have the right knowledge.
- I am too lazy to change.

If you feel despair in your attempt to achieve your ideal health and resonate with some of the above statements, you must start challenging them now. I know many successful people in the area of finances or relationships who are struggling with weight and health issues, and they have some very negative beliefs about their health.

Exercise: What other reasons/beliefs can you add to this list that keep you stuck at your current weight/health level?

By entertaining these beliefs in our lives, we are disconnected from our real personal power. And from the disempowered state:

- Instead of looking after your health with nourishing food and drinks, you may choose cheap takeaways and fast food or overeating of 'healthy' food.
- You punish yourself by drinking excessively (associated with dangerous behaviours like impulsivity, and being prone to accidents) or smoking.
- You may prioritize your work over your sleep, staying up late to complete other responsibilities.

These are just learned limiting beliefs that keep us stuck. There is enough evidence in the world that optimum health is always a possibility – no matter what your personal history has been or your income level or if you are man or woman or if you believe you have the resources or not.

So, I welcome you to choose to believe that:

"I am in the process of achieving my dream health, and the process of making a positive lifestyle change is easy and joyful."

If you wish to see positive changes in your health, you may like to change these negative beliefs to more empowering ones.

The reverse of the above negative beliefs:

- My past does not equal my future; I can achieve a lighter body.
- I am finding newer ways to prepare and enjoy healthy food that nourishes my body and mind.
- I am enjoying a balance in all areas of my life.
- I am discovering new approaches that will suit my unique body and give me positive results.
- It's never too late to start.
- I am discovering new avenues for success.
- I am in the process of making positive changes.

CHAPTER 4

Self-worth and Deservability

"I am worthy and deserving of incredible
and vibrant health."
—Pranita Salunke

Louise Hay, a pioneering expert, and author of *Heal Your Life* suggests that going beyond the surface-level limiting beliefs mentioned initially, there is a bigger problem – our deep-seated fears, and feelings of:

- I am not good enough,
- A lack of self-worth,
- A lack of self-love,
- A lack of deservability.

With her teachings, especially affirmations and mirror techniques, Louise Hay has assisted millions of people healing from many diseases by encouraging them to love, approve and accept themselves before making progress in their desired goals.

Let us get inspiration from her wisdom and start declaring our worthiness and self-acceptance.

Exercises to improve self-worth and self-love

1. Mirrorwork:

First thing in the morning and every time you pass the mirror, look deep into your eyes and say:

'Your name,' I love you and accept you as you are right now.

Make a list of your strengths: a list of what qualities you love or like about yourself. If you are unsure, ask your friends or trusted advisors what they find most appealing in you. You may be pleasantly surprised.

List your strengths

Compliment and appreciate all your positives.
Your beauty: write your favourite features.
Your wisdom.
All the skills you possess.
Loving relationships you share with others: your spouse, family, your work colleagues.
Your personality traits: for example, kindness, compassion, creativity, etc.
Adventures you have experienced.
Your career, business success.

Keep reminding and reinforcing your strengths throughout your day and every time you pass the mirror.

Exercise: List your positive aspects, strengths, successes.

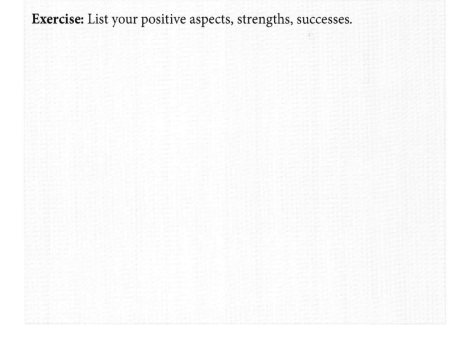

2. Affirmations to improve your self-worth:

Repeat these positive statements with feeling in the morning and at night. Pick any ideas which resonate with you the most or create your own inspiring ones.

- I love, approve, and accept myself for who I am.
- I radiate and receive love and respect.
- I am loved and respected wherever I go.
- I am unique in my talents and abilities and do not need validation from others.
- I deserve all that is good.
- I am grateful for all the beautiful things in my life.
- I am full of loving, healthy, positive, and prosperous thoughts, which eventually convert into my life experiences.
- I am solution driven. Every problem is a chance to grow.
- I am never alone in my pursuit of success. The universe supports me in expected and unexpected ways.
- Only I am responsible for making my choices and decisions.
- I love the person I am becoming.
- I am giving priority to my desires.
- Every moment brings us a choice, and I choose happiness no matter what my circumstances.
- I am flexible and flowing, open to new experiences.
- I think positively and expect the best.
- I am aware of my strength and act with confidence.
- Life is beautiful and rewarding.
- The universe blesses me with health, happiness, and abundance.
- I appreciate the things I have. I rejoice in the love I receive.
- I am courageous. My eyes reflect the strength of my soul.
- I am cheerful and optimistic. The universe conspires to make me successful.
- I am passionate about what I do, and my enthusiasm reflects that in my work.
- I attract positive and helping people in my life.

- I am open to meeting people and create positive and supportive relationships.
- I radiate love and inspire people.
- I am calm and peaceful.
- I take time to enjoy the little joys of life.

I have created a meditation to strengthen your self-worth, especially about achieving your health goals.

Enjoy the video by visiting https://pranitavitality.com/video/

CHAPTER 5

Release Negativity and Embrace Positivity

Another mindset limitation that hinders our progress towards achieving our health goals is cultivating negative emotions towards ourselves and others. Many physical diseases have roots in these negative emotions – such as anger, resentment, or guilt. When you release them from your consciousness, you lay the foundations for a healthy, happy and fulfilling life of your desire.

My personal experience of being in abusive relationships in childhood and early adulthood made me very angry towards those who abused me; it also made me fearful of the future. The cumulative effect of this emotional state affected my health and manifested in digestive issues.

Doing a lot of inner work and meditations, I realised that the negativity I harboured was harming me more than it affected 'them' in any way. THEY treated me the way they did because of their knowledge and experience; the fear and lack of love they had themselves. The child in them was starved of love and approval, and they couldn't give me anything that they didn't have. The path to my healing and wellness started with the readiness to let go and forgive the past.

Could you look at your negative life experiences from this similar perspective?

Are you ready to forgive yourself and those who have hurt you?

Are you ready to let go of your past traumas?

Exercise:

Identifying negative emotions:

- What are some of the negative feelings you regularly experience that are keeping you stuck in the past?

- Name them: Guilt/shame/anger/resentment/blame…

- Towards who and why? Self/Others?

*"Forgiveness and love are two secrets to
your holistic healing."*
—Pranita Salunke

Forgiveness Exercises

These are some of the ways you can approach the forgiveness of old hurts.

1. Physical release:

Negative emotions of anger, frustration, and resentment are stored in your body at a cellular level. Some intense physical activity is a great way to release that negativity. While keeping your intention on the experience or person you feel anger towards, use all your force while doing the activity and ask yourself, "What is it about this that makes me angry?"

You may experience sadness, tears, and after all that, a feeling of lightness in your heart.

You could try:
Screaming in the woods, jogging, running, swimming, boxing or even hitting a pillow.

2. Be willing to forgive:

Know that learnings from difficult experiences make you a much better evolved human being.

The past is there to teach some lessons that our soul needs to learn. I know that I had to learn the lessons of forgiveness, hence unconsciously I chose to be in those abusive relationships.

It does not mean that you acknowledge and accept the unfair treatment from those people.

But you are willing to forgive their ignorance at that time. They would have done better, if they knew better.

3. Forgive and set yourself free:

You can do this step in a few different ways:

Visualise

You can close your eyes and visualise the person (or yourself) and say:

I am angry/sad/hurtful for you doing this …… (actions that hurt you) …… to me.

But I know that it is limiting my progress in my life.

Thank you for sharing this soul lesson with me …… (write the lesson you learned).

I am sorry for causing you to distress knowingly or unknowingly.
I entirely forgive myself for allowing this experience.
I entirely forgive you (name) for your actions.

I now bless myself and you with love and gratitude.

You are free, and I am free.

I am open to experience a beautiful life.

4. Write a letter:

Write a letter to the person who you need to forgive. Write all about how their behaviour made you feel, the consequences of that you are currently experiencing. Write about what alternative treatment you would have preferred from them. How could they right the wrong they have done to you so that you can forgive them? Vividly imagine that they are actively listening and are expressing their apology to you. You could write about how it feels to hear "sorry" from them. You are now compassionately accepting their apology and forgiving them for their past behaviour. You may note tears as you are expressing your heart in your letter; let them flow freely.

Embrace Positivity

"Appreciation inspires optimum health and happiness."
—Pranita Salunke

Love and appreciation are two of the purest emotions that enhance our sense of well-being and contribute to healing. Condemning, berating, and criticising our looks and worrying about our health conditions will only enhance disharmony within us. It will make us procrastinate or lead us to make excuses for not taking action for our health goals. Instead, when we love and appreciate the numerous gifts we already possess, we allow an abundance of health, energy, vitality, and anything else we desire to flow into our life.

Be content in the now.

If you have been dealing with health issues for a long time, you may think that you don't have anything to appreciate, but that is not true.

You can always start appreciating what is working in other areas of your life - for example, your wonderful family, parents, friends, the love and connection you share. Or your work, the money you earn, and the freedom it provides to you, enjoying meals, travel, and buying things of your choice.

Or you could appreciate non-tangible things like the beautiful sunshine you are enjoying, birds singing, or you could appreciate the air around you - without the air, we can't breathe, breath is life, without which we can't survive. What a beautiful privilege we have!

Appreciation of small things enhances our perspective on life and gives us internal power to sustain positive changes in our lives, including transforming our lifestyle.

Exercise:

Make your list of appreciations/gratitude:

I have created this Gratitude visualisation for you – you can listen to it here: https://pranitavitality.com/video/

SECTION 2

Lifestyle Strategies

"A positive lifestyle is key to your ultimate transformation!"
—Pranita Salunke

CHAPTER 6

Nourishment

"Let food be thy medicine and medicine be thy food."
—Hippocrates

Good food energizes our body with nutrition and nourishes our soul and its fundamental objectives of giving us nutrition. For many centuries, dining has been viewed as a multisensory ritual for connection, an experience we share with loving family and friends or savour it ourselves. I still remember my mother's cooking, which was unbeatable in its taste even compared with world-renowned chefs, because it was made of pure love for me. I am sure you can relate to this experience. Even in the professional world, the term 'breaking the bread' is used to strengthen relationships with business partners, clients, and employees. This chapter aims to inspire you to enjoy the food that is gifted to us by nature.

Food is medicine. Decades ago, there were no diet products, nutritionists or dieticians, yet chronic diseases like type 2 diabetes were not common. People chose food close to nature and savoured it with their loved ones. Many ancient cultures still eat according to these principles, and therefore they enjoy a long and healthy life.

As we discussed in the first chapter, society has had a role in creating lifestyle diseases – the modern, highly competitive, fast-paced culture has negatively transformed our eating habits and preferences.

Many conflicting academic studies are published every day, promoting the importance of one type of food or another. In contrast, the very next day, another research banishes that same food element, which adds to our existing confusion.

Considering this modern-day conflict, what should the optimum eating style be to ensure we not only enjoy the food that nourishes our body and keeps chronic diseases at bay, but also energizes our mind and lightens our spirit?

The answer is simple.

Rather than looking for outside help, tune in to your body to know what nourishment it is really seeking and simply feed it.

It sounds simple in principle, but how would it work in practice?

For any prevention strategies designed to control chronic diseases and enjoy a slender body, a significant shift from a typical 'Western diet' is imperative.

This chapter aims not to propose another 'diet' plan and offer a specific balance of carbohydrates, fats, proteins, vitamins, and minerals. There are excellent books written on these topics already by experts. I hope instead to equip you with an arsenal of healthy eating principles that have the power to prevent and control chronic conditions.

When incorporated as a part of your daily life, these healthy eating principles will help you to:

- Balance your blood sugar and reduce underlying chronic inflammation that is a precursor for many chronic diseases. It will assist you to reverse or control diabetes, reduce excess weight, normalise high blood pressure.

Enjoying this healthy eating style, you will also:

- Gain incredible energy for all the essential areas of your life.
- Your skin will glow from inside.
- It will also give you the pleasure of savouring delicious, nourishing, and hearty food.

We will discuss healthy eating principles for heart health, supported by scientific studies, and integrate them with ancient holistic philosophy based on Ayurveda and mindfulness.

Nourishment for a Healthy and Happy Heart: Remove, Replace and Rejuvenate Principle.

I believe our body is a beautiful vessel that blossoms from inside out with nourishing and energising food. However, if the vessel is already filled with unhealthy food (a.k.a debris), even the best eating guidance will not help us to create the optimum healthy heart and vibrant life we desire.

The first step is always to clear the space by REMOVING foods and drinks that are harmful to the health of our body and mind. We then can REPLACE that space with natural, healing, heart-warming foods and REJUVENATE our cells with optimum micronutrients and superfoods. It also means optimizing our environment, so we overcome emotional eating and take joy in savouring healthy and happy heart meals with our loved ones.

Remove

Learning from a successful author and world-class organising expert Marie Kondo could be of immense value when considering our eating habits. Her teachings inform us that if we wish to live in a beautiful, organised environment, we have to get rid of items that do not "spark joy" in our lives, decluttering, unused belongings or things that create stress instead of value. Similarly, if we want to "spark energy and health" in our lives, we have to start removing foods that are harmful to our body and mind.

We have to remove the following pro-inflammatory foods (food that creates inflammation and diseases) before our body can absorb nutritious food.

1. Modern 'convenient' food:

With global growth in 'Western Lifestyle,' the art of eating has been reduced to a mere act of consuming calories to fuel our body with a low-quality diet of processed, packaged, and refined products. These foods are often less expensive to purchase and heavily marketed by their manufacturers, making them convenient to consume by all of us.

When you are busy at work and have forgotten to bring a packed lunch, it is easy to go to the supermarket, get a meal deal of a packaged sandwich, fruit juice, and a crisp packet full of salt. Result? A sudden increase in sugar levels that gives temporary satisfaction but causes long-term damage.

Refined carbohydrates like white bread, white pasta, white sugar, sugary juices, high sodium, unhealthy fats, and sugar give us temporary pleasure but create insulin imbalance and inflammation in our body. The danger of these foods is evident with the growing rate of lifestyle-related diseases across the globe.

Examples of refined food to remove:

- White bread, white pasta, white sugars.
- Sweetened beverages including sodas, juices, sports drinks, excessive teas, and coffees.
- Packaged biscuits, muffins, cakes.
- Instant pizza, burgers, pasta and noodles.
- Processed meats and sausages.
- Bread, breakfast foods and other products made from cereals and grains.
- Takeaway foods like fish and chips.

2. Sugar: Sugar stimulates the reward centre of the brain and releases 'pleasure' hormones, making it as addictive and harmful to your body as any 'drug'.(1) High sugar causes an imbalance in insulin levels and your metabolism, which in turn leads to an increase in belly fat and obesity. Sugar in our system releases inflammatory markers such as cytokinin, a precursor for many chronic diseases.

A scientific review by the British Cardiovascular Society published in 2017 demonstrates a close link between high sugar and heart disease by creating insulin imbalance leading to obesity, type 2 diabetes, cancer and dementia.(2)

3. Craving for savoury/salty food: One of the reasons refined packaged foods are dangerous is that they contain too much salt. Over time, overeating sodium can increase your risk of high blood pressure, a significant risk factor for CVD and cancer.

Joint British Society's guideline for CVD prevention: <u>less than 5g of salt.</u>

Swap high salt with herbs and spices. One way to get over the craving for salty or savoury food is to enjoy a citrusy zing with lemons or oranges, use aromatic herbs like basil and coriander, and flavour your wholesome meal with tangy spices like crushed black pepper or Julian ginger. I have found fresh olives help me to limit the craving for savoury packaged food. Try it yourself.

4. 'Low calorie' foods: fact or fiction?

For years, we have been led to believe that healthy weight = calorie in < calorie out. I think this is not true. Your body will metabolise a 100-calorie vanilla ice-cream scoop or Coke differently to 100 calories of apples, carrots, or oranges. One is loaded with sugar, artificial preservatives and colours, while others are full of natural vitamins, minerals, fibres, and phytonutrients.

Dr Dariush Mozzaffarian, a well-respected doctor and epidemiologist suggests in his scientific review that focusing on calories can be misleading as not all calories are created equal in the relation to weight gain and obesity. (3)

Counting calories is also a psychologically tiring experience. The constant focus and worry about knowing the exact calories of each mouthful you are consuming is draining, and it is not part of a sustainable lifestyle.

Suggestion:

Tune in your body.

Eat in response to 'real hunger'.

Eat intuitively and be mindful of the source of your meal rather than counting calories (more about mindful eating discussed later in the chapter).

5. Low or zero-sugar food

Food manufacturers are inventing newer low-sugar products continuously. For many decades, we have fallen prey to the temptation of being (or looking) like attractive models shown on these food commercials. But it is an illusion. To make these low or zero-sugar foods, manufacturers replace fat and sugar in real food with food additives like corn syrup and cellulose (obtained from wood – a cheaper resource) to make them edible. These additives are linked with weight gain and severe digestive issues.(4)

There is a disagreement within the academic field about artificial sweeteners' safety like aspartame (an ingredient in many diet products). A few researchers have shown its link with increased cancer risks including, lymphoma and leukaemia in the past.(5) Although the FDA (The United States Food and Drug Administration) disagrees with these studies and has approved this for use as a sweetener, on the premise that because it is about 200 times sweeter than usual sugar, people may use it less. (6)

I believe that if we can avoid these artificial sugars by learning to enjoy natural food, why take the risk?

Furthermore, as sweeteners like saccharine or aspartame are up to 200 times sweeter than sugar, they also increase the craving for the same products – making us drink and eat even more of those foods and ultimately making us FAT. Many slimming products, shakes/liquids are meant to replace your meals have fewer calories, but a higher number of artificial sweeteners, additives, and emulsifiers that lead to inflammation and disruption in your gut lining. Considering its detrimental effect on digestion, weight, and overall health, are these types of diets and low-sugar/fat foods worth investing our money and energy?

In her book, 'Feeding you Lies', *New York Times'* best-selling author, Vani Hari, goes in depth to bust some 'diet' myths. It is a good read if you need to know the science behind all the fad diets.(4) For now, I would encourage you to keep away from the temptation of adding white sugar, artificial replacements, or any 'diet' products to your eating plan.

6. Commercial Trans fats

Small amounts of trans fats occur naturally in ruminants like beef, lamb, and dairy products. Although natural trans fats are produced in the gut of some grazing animals (such as cattle and sheep), the commercial trans fats are dangerous and should not be consumed.

Artificial trans fats are processed fats, made to enhance food flavours, make them cheaper, and increase shelf-life. They are found in margarine, processed foods, fried foods like doughnuts, French fries, takeaways, and chicken nuggets.

However, the so-called 'benefits' of these fats come with serious health risks. Academic guidelines worldwide warn us against consuming trans fats, which are strongly linked with the development of type 2 diabetes and heart diseases. For every 2% of calories from trans fat consumed daily, the risk of heart disease rises by 23%.(7)

Trans fats increase 'bad' cholesterol including Low-Density Lipoprotein, (LDL); Very Low-Density Lipoprotein (VLDL) and Triglycerides. At the same time, they reduce levels of 'good cholesterol' High-Density Lipoprotein (HDL).(8,9,10)

Ways to REMOVE trans fats from your diet

Food labels: Don't be seduced by the 0 g of the trans-fat label; it might still contain trans fats. Look and avoid ingredients listed on a food package as: 'partially hydrogenated oils'.

Some ingredients do not need to be labelled as trans fats according to the FDA, even if they contain trace amounts of trans fats: some refined oils, artificial flavours and colours, monoglycerides and diglycerides converted as triglycerides in our body and usually labelled as 'emulsifiers'.

Simple ways to remove trans fats are:

- Avoid processed, packaged, preserved food and takeaways.
- Try baking, broiling, grilling, or steaming. These cooking methods do not add extra fat.
- In a restaurant, don't be afraid to ask and see the labels of oils used in your food preparation.

7. External substances

Smoking: tobacco consumption of any kind, including second-hand smoking and excess alcohol consumption, leads to an increased risk of CVD. These activities are also carcinogenic (increased risk of cancer) in their nature. These are toxic substances that lead to a chronic inflammatory response in your body. Smoking increases the risk of nearly all cardiovascular diseases.(11,12)

A 30-year-long public health research investigated the effect of these two harmful behaviours (smoking and excessive drinking) when combined. The researcher found that compared with never-smokers, men who both smoked and drank 15+ units/week had the highest risk (2.71 times) of dying prematurely; that is before the age of 65.(13)

Tips to overcome the addiction:

- Seek professional support to overcome the habits of smoking and excessive drinking (use a professional trained in health behaviour changes).
- In the early stages of making positive changes, limit your contacts/associations who indulge in these unhealthy behaviours, and seek encouragement from supportive family and friends.

- Improve your overall positive lifestyle, getting active, and drinking more water.
- Follow the lifestyle advice and health behavioural changes discussed in this book.
- Keep your motivation high by reading success stories online and knowing you could achieve these results yourself.

8. Gut health food intolerances

"You are not what you eat, but how much you digest."
—Pranita Salunke

In the current world, many factors are responsible for the ever-growing incidences of food allergies and gut intolerances, a phenomenon which was rare decades ago. I believe, the interplay of many factors is creating this rise, such as the quality of soil and seeds of the grains, packaging of the food products, sedentary lifestyle, increasing stress levels and our ability or inability to process that stress.

These gut intolerances result in an increase in systemic inflammation, which leads to chronic disease, gut disorders, and, in general, poor quality of life.

Some of the symptoms of food intolerances are:

- Joint pain
- Eczema
- Bloating, stomach pain or colicky symptoms
- Change in appearance of your stools, etc.

Although intolerances are specific to the individual, there are some common culprits that we need to be mindful of:

- Monosodium glutamate (MSG)
- Caffeine
- Alcohol
- Artificial sweeteners

- Histamine (found in Quorn, mushrooms, pickled and cured foods, and alcoholic drinks)
- Toxins, viruses, bacteria or parasites that have contaminated food
- Artificial food colours, preservatives or flavour enhancers
- Gluten
- Eggs
- Peanuts or tree nuts
  Reference:14

Solution

To identify which specific food is creating symptoms, you may choose to get a laboratory food sensitivity test. However, another way to determine the sensitivity is by the following:

1. Elimination diet:

- Keep food and thought diary (Resources) to find the thought/food pattern or a particular food item because of your symptoms.
- Eliminate the food source for 3–4 weeks, before gradually re-introducing it back to your diet.
- If the symptoms persist, continue to eliminate that food.
- If you are worried that you may be missing out on vital nutrition, seek support from a health professional.
- Support your gut health by the advice discussed in the 'Replace' section.

2. Mindfulness: Meditation and breathing exercises, ss described in this book, will help you calm your gut before a meal, making it a more nourishing experience as opposed to creating stress-related intolerances.

9. Toxicity

On a positive note, we as a society are becoming more conscious of eating healthy food. But despite our best intentions, parasiticides and herbicides that cover our food, and toxic food packaging have a significant role in today's rising epidemic of chronic diseases.

In her book, *Feeding You Lies,* food activist Vani Hari, lifts the veil on many hidden ingredients, food lobbying, and even manipulated academic research that influences policies and our eating behaviour. Considering the importance of this element, in the table below, I would enlist some of the harmful and toxic chemicals in our food and environment so that you can make a conscious choice to avoid them for achieving optimum health). However, I would encourage you to read above book to get an in-depth insight into this topic.(4)

Our skin is the largest organ, that consumes chemical toxins from the environment, skincare, makeup, and personal care products. Choose wisely. The list below is not exhaustive, as there will no doubt be newer tricks invented by manufacturers to make their products appear 'healthy'! (Be mindful when you shop).

Remember, we need to be mindful that our skin is the largest organ, which consumes chemical toxins from the environment and food with artificial flavours and or additives.

Category	Specific agents	Action
Food additives	Sugar, high fructose corn syrup, saccharine, sucralose, aspartame.	Be conscious while shopping and choose products without the above ingredients
	Canola and vegetable oils, chemically refined soybean oils.	Food should be simple: if you don't understand an ingredient, it is possible that it is not safe for you.
	MSG.	
	Mono and diglycerides.	Choose dairy products from ethical sources and organic farmers.
	Partially hydrogenated oils.	
	Products with Genetically Modified Organism (GMO).	Follow the guidance of nourishing food and drinks discussed in this book, by which you can resist the temptations of fast food and beverages with these additives.
	Emulsifiers such as cellulose gel and cellulose gums. They damage gut microbiome, increase systemic	

Category	Specific agents	Action
	inflammation, leading to digestive disorders and obesity and metabolic syndrome. Carrageenan are linked with cancer and inflammation in intestine. Diet shakes because they are filled with artificial sweeteners and additives – which lead to imbalances of hunger hormones, increased appetite and therefore fat production. Hormone-treated dairy and dairy products.	
Pesticides and herbicides – in the environment and sprayed over food packaging like plastic and food containers. They are linked to the release of obesogenic chemicals (which are linked with many metabolic diseases).	Some of them are: BHT and Nitrates.	Read the labels and remove them from your lifestyle.
Sugar with alternative names.	High fructose corn syrup, saccharine, 76-sucralose.	Remove the products with these ingredients.
Environmental toxins are linked with insulin resistance which leads to obesity and diabetes.	Some of them are BPA, phthalates: found in packaging, plastics, plastic water bottles. vinyl flooring, detergents and cosmetics, air-fresheners and household cleaning products.	Avoid food that comes in plastic packaging as much as you can. Use freshly cut tomatoes, vegetables, fruits; hand soak pulses and legumes overnight instead of buying canned products.

Category	Specific agents	Action
	Synthetic pesticides found in non-organic produce, grains and meat products.	Choose organic produce or shop at your local farmers' market.
		Soak and wash your fruits and vegetables thoroughly.
		Buy organic skin-care, make-up and home products.
		Switch to home-filtered water. Invest in a high-quality water filter or buy water with glass containers.
		If time permits, create DIY home cleaning products: there are many online resources available to inspire and guide you with this goal should you wish to do so.
Food containers While cooking, these chemicals seep through our food and are linked with many conditions, (such as PFOA linked to thyroid diseases, etc.)	Pans and pots made with aluminium or chemicals such as PFOA (perfluorooctanoic acid) found in non-sticks and cans.	Use pots and pans made with cast iron, earthenware (used in many traditional cultures including India) ceramic, or stainless steel.

Reference (4)

Do all these changes sound overwhelming? Maybe at first. Therefore, I encourage you, before moving on to the next stage of healthy eating (replace and rejuvenate) to take stock of your current food habits and environmental toxins that could be damaging your health. It helps to make a 3 to 7-day diary to see any triggers and patterns in your food and health symptoms (you could download the 3 -day lifestyle diary here: https://pranitavitality.com/resources/)

Make a conscious decision to REMOVE unhealthy ingredients from your life. Start with removing one thing at a time and then slowly build up your momentum, until you feel confident that you have created the space for nourishing food that supports your health goals.

Replace and Rejuvenate:

Congratulations on removing low-quality food from your life. Now you have ample space to get nourished with superior-quality products that really can create optimum health and happiness.

Just remember this is not a diet plan. I am offering my experience of healthy eating and bringing more consciousness into the way we eat. Of course, when you incorporate this eating style, it will give you the best protection against chronic diseases, including cardiovascular disease, lifestyle-related cancer, and it will also assist you in maintaining your brain health.

With this knowledge, I encourage you to make the necessary adjustments to your eating style and, rather than sticking to this only for a limited time only, make these principles your 'new way of being'!

The Protective Power of Plant Foods:

The rainbow colours of plant-based foods, fruits, vegetables, seeds, nuts, legumes, and whole grains are bursting with the body's essential building blocks. Amino acids, complex carbohydrates (essential for slow release of sugar) and bio-active compounds called phytonutrients are present in plant foods to give us the burst of vitamins, minerals, and antioxidants necessary for energy, nourishment and recovery from diseases. The health benefits of a plant-based diet go beyond improving your heart health; it also protects us against cancer, brain ageing, dementia, improves sexual health, gives us glowing skin, and youthful energy.

One of the well-researched eating styles, incorporating the above food components, is the 'Mediterranean diet'. The Mediterranean diet is based on eating plenty of fruits, vegetables, whole grains, legumes, and fats from oily fish, olive oil, nuts, and only moderate alcohol consumption.

Various studies worldwide have shown the protective effect of a strict Mediterranean diet against CVD, cancers, and Alzheimer's disease. A significant hallmark study has shown a 75% reduction in dying from all causes, including cardiovascular diseases and cancer, among people who ate a diet with a higher Mediterranean score (compared to those who ate food with a lower Mediterranean score). (15)

Another public health study links the Mediterranean diet with improvement in functional abilities, even in older people. The survey conducted on nearly 1500 French men and women concluded that the higher the Mediterranean score, the more improved functional performance and the less chance of being disabled. These findings are relevant because as we get older, maintaining our functions, daily activities, brain function, and work performance is directly linked with our dignity and quality of life. (16) A hallmark study, the Lyon Diet Heart Study also showed that a higher Mediterranean score is associated with a lesser risk of cardiovascular complications in people with established heart diseases. (17)

Fibres from fruits and vegetables serve as prebiotics, feeding nutrients to our gut organisms, producing pro-biotics, and more diverse gut flora maintaining healthy digestion. Rich polyphenols found in olives, green and black teas, as well as herbs like rosemary, thyme, mint and dark chocolate are linked with improvement in overall health, energy and they also have anti-ageing properties.

The following table illustrates the importance of a rainbow of plant and vegetable colours for your health.

Make a conscious effort to choose different colours of fruits and vegetables in your diet.

	Phyto nutrients	Benefits	Found in
Reds	Lycopene. Anthocyanin, ellagic acid, Vitamin C.	Prevent heart and lung diseases, cancer, vision loss.	Tomatoes. Strawberries. Goji berries. Red vegetables, red cabbage
Orange	Carotenes, Beta-Carotenes, bio-flavonoids, beta cryptothanxin.	Provides vitamin A, Improves immunity and eye health.	Oranges. Yellow fruits and vegetables – like yellow pepper, carrots, orange, mangoes, grapefruit, corns.
Green	Lutein, chlorophyll, indoles, folate, nitrate, Vitamin .K	Improves immunity. Detoxing. Anti-cancer. Blood and bone health.	Leafy greens, sprouted grass, broccoli, cabbage, kelp, peas, cucumber, avocado, asparagus.
Whites	Allyl sulphide Antioxidants	Anti-inflammatory. Improves heart health and gives protection against cancer.	Onions, garlics, banana, cauliflower, potato, garlic, turnips.
Blues	Anthocyanins Resveratrol	Support healthy aging and brain health. Balance hormones.	Blueberries, aubergine, grapes, red wine (1-2 units per day max. If you don't drink wine, it is absolutely fine, just choose other sources of blue.)

Reference: 18, 19, 20

*Dark chocolate also gives us essential antioxidants. Ensure you use a small amount with a higher percentage of cocoa.

Practical steps to ensure how we can get a maximum rainbow diet:

1. Motivate and involve all family members to enjoy a rainbow of fruits and vegetables.

2. Enjoy healthy snacks of fruits, vegetables, and nuts instead of reaching for savoury crisps or sugary cookies.

   A few snack ideas:

   Veg crudities (carrots, celery, peppers, cucumber) with hummus or nut butter; green olives.

3. Add herbs and lemon to make vegetables zingier and more palatable.

Recipe suggestion using fruits and vegetables

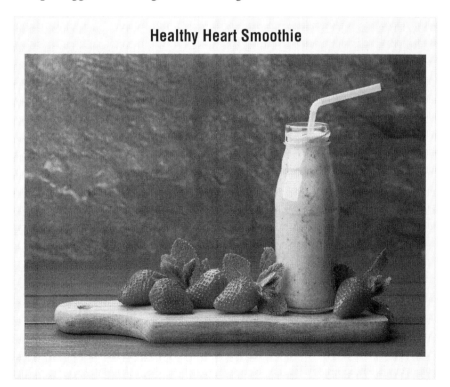

Healthy Heart Smoothie

Your heart will thank you for the nourishing nutrients from these yummy fruits and vegetables. Mix and match any fruits and vegetables you have available. If your digestion cannot handle too many fibres in your smoothies, feel free to extract the nutrients with juicing (except the avocado).

Adjust the portion to suit your personal taste.

- 50% green vegetables of your choice: lettuce, spinach, kale (approximately 1 cup)
- 1 teaspoon of toasted flax or chia or sunflower seeds or 5-10 soaked[4] walnuts
- ½ cup blueberries/strawberries
- 1 apple or ½ banana (depending on the availability)
- Juice of half a lemon (optional)

Fill your smoothie maker jar with these ingredients and whisk with some water to make a delicious, colourful drink, which, if you savour slowly, could be regarded as a light meal.

**The approximate amount is indicated here, use your intuition and common sense to choose the ingredients and portions.

Wholesome Carbohydrates

Carbohydrates (carbs) are the essential building blocks of nourishment. I strongly disagree with the modern-age NO-carb diet advice for weight loss or diabetes control. I believe wholesome carbs give us various vitamins and nutrients. They also balance our insulin levels, providing energy and feelings of satiety (so that we don't keep eating for hours).

---

[4] The process of toasting enhances the flavour, and soaking seeds and nuts improves their nutrient quality and aids in their digestion.

I tested the no-grain/no-carb approach for a few weeks as part of an experiment for this book. What I noted was that my craving for sugary and high-fat foods shot through the roof and I had to fight to maintain my weight. At the end of this experiment, I realised that this approach for weight-loss or disease control is limiting and unsustainable in the long run. I would encourage you to choose and enjoy a small portion of wholesome carbs with your meals.

Healthy carbs include:

- Grains, for example, rice (red/brown/purple/black), amaranth, teff or quinoa.
- Root vegetables such as sweet potatoes, turnips, or swede.

These are all eaten across many traditional cultures like Asia, Latin America, Africa.

A Note on Gluten

In recent years, gluten-containing grains like wheat have been linked with inflammation, coeliac disease, and digestive issues. If you are experiencing any of these conditions, it is better to stay clear of the grains containing gluten. However, do not choose gluten-free replacements as they may often have unwanted additives or substitutes, which can cause more harm than good. Instead, it is best to opt for some of the wholesome carbs listed above. When we eat wholesome carbs in a limited quantity, we get all the benefits of nutrients derived from that particular food without spiking our blood glucose.

The next section will educate you on the effect of different carbohydrates in balancing your blood glucose and assist you with weight loss and diabetes control.

Wholesome Risotto with Chicken or Lentil and Chickpeas.

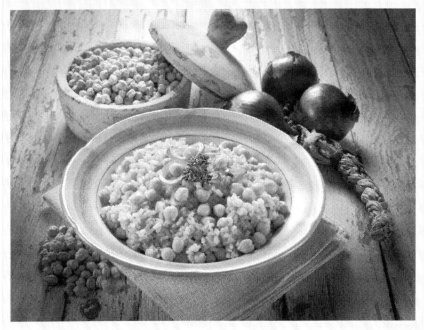

When made with wholesome carbs such as bulgur wheat or brown rice, an Italian dish would suit your taste buds and your waistline.

Ingredients: serves approx. 2

- 1 cup bulgur wheat or brown rice: soaked (for 2 hours) and rinsed
- ½ cup lentils and ½ cup chickpeas
- or two chicken breasts, diced to 1-inch cubes, seasoned with salt and pepper
- 1 red onion, finely chopped
- 1–2 garlic cloves, minced
- Olive oil
- Salt
- Pepper

- 1 red chilli: deseeded and chopped (optional)
- 1 red pepper, deseeded and chopped
- Chopped herbs: parsley, thyme, coriander
- 1 bay leaf
- 1–2 cups of water
- 1 cube of vegetable stock (optional, ensure no harmful ingredients in it)
- 2 lemon wedges to serve

Preparation:

1. In a saucepan (preferably made with iron/copper), cook chicken with a little olive oil until browned on all sides. Remove the cooked chicken from the pan.
2. Or if you are choosing a vegetarian option, cook chickpeas and lentils according to package instructions.
3. In a saucepan, sauté the chopped onion and garlic for a few minutes, taking care not to burn it.
4. Add a bay leaf, bulgur wheat or brown rice, and red pepper. Cover with water and let it simmer until cooked.
5. Stir in either chicken or lentils and chickpeas and sauté for another few minutes, and let it slowly cook for 10 mins and then cover with a lid.
6. Season with chopped herbs, salt and pepper, before serving with lemon wedges and a pinch of love.

Suggestion: you can swap chicken, lentils, or chickpeas with tofu or halloumi cheese to add variety to your dinner.

The Glycaemic Index

The Glycaemic Index (GI) is the effect that different carbohydrates have on your glucose level. Low GI Complex CHO has low GI; they produce only small fluctuations in our blood glucose and insulin level and give you a feeling of satisfaction.

Eating Low GI food has long-term benefits on your health – weight management, reducing the risk of heart disease, improving lipid (cholesterol) levels – and offers better diabetes control by improving insulin sensitivity.

GI of different food groups:

	Low GI	Medium GI	High GI
Grains	Wholegrain, granary, corn tortilla, brown rice.	Pitta, chapatti, couscous, basmati rice.	Baguette, bagel, white wholemeal bread, white rice.
Legumes	Chickpeas, kidney beans, lentils, soybeans.		
Cereals	Oat-based (porridge, muesli), bran-rich, muesli, millet porridge.	Cereal bars	Wheat or maize based (cornflakes, Weetabix).
Fruit	Berries, oranges, lemons, apples.	Dried fruit, banana, pineapple, mangoes.	Fruit juice, watermelon, lychees.
Vegetables	All green and salad. Vegetables, carrots, yam, new potatoes in skin.	Sweet potato, sweetcorn, beetroot, boiled old potatoes, chips.	Pumpkin, parsnips, jacket potatoes.
Dairy/non-dairy	Plain yogurt, milk, soymilk.		Flavoured yogurt.
Sugar	Fructose.	Sucrose, honey.	Glucose.

Reference: 21, 22

Glycaemic Load:

The size of blood sugar fluctuation is also affected by the ripeness of food, the method of cooking and portion size, and food combination, which is measured as Glycaemic Load (GL).

The GL of eating three vegetable stews and a Sunday roast will be much higher than eating a small portion for mid-week lunch.

Suggestions to reduce the glycaemic load:

Analyse the GL of your entire meal and see if you can reduce foods that have a high GI; increase foods with a low GI and control your portion size. Often, raised portions are related to emotional eating. Suggestions described in the section of 'Emotional Eating' will help you to overcome this challenge (if any).

Healthy Fats

Fats are essential for the optimum performance of human cells, hormone production, and our nervous system's efficient functioning. Therefore, the right fats are critical for maintaining your optimum health and preventing dementia, depression, and chronic diseases.

As our body is unable to make fats itself, these must be eaten via food sources. But the key to prevent or control chronic diseases and stay at a healthy weight is to consume the right balance of fats in the right amounts.

Right Fats vs. Wrong Fats:

Omega-3 fats, which are found in foods such as oily fish and flaxseed, are anti-inflammatory in nature. However, during the industrial revolution, we learned to extract oils from seeds, beans, and vegetables into refined oils filled with poly-unsaturated fatty acids with omega six fats. (23) A high percentage of Omega-6 in our body leads to inflammation, reducing the beneficiary effect of anti-inflammatory Omega-3 fats.

For many decades, well-respected authorities' guidance was to replace saturated fats found in animal sources like milk or butter with vegetable oils filled with polyunsaturated fatty acids – PUFA. (23) As a result, our current diet is significantly high in Omega-6 fats.

Animals (chicken, sheep, etc.) are now being fed with Omega-6 filled seeds rather than feeding on natural grass. This is further adding to the mayhem and increases the body's Omega-6 content for people who consume animal products. This shift in our eating style has increased the Omega-6: Omega-3 ratio in our body.

This shift could be one factor contributing to higher occurrences of chronic diseases in our society. (24,25) To reverse this damage, we have to work towards reversing this ratio. This means eating more fats that give us anti-inflammatory Omega-3 and fewer fats with pro-inflammatory Omega-6.

The findings from hallmark scientific research support this statement. Randomised control trials (RCT) are considered gold standards in clinical research, as people are randomly divided into different interventions to minimise statistical distortion.

The Lyon Heart Study, a RCT, demonstrated that when participants consumed significantly fewer fats from Omega-6 and higher fats from Omega-3, the heart attack rate and death from all causes, including stroke and cancer, were reduced by a significant 70 per cent!!! (26)

Another RCT, PREDIMED, successfully demonstrated the heart protection benefits of eating healthy fats. The study published in the *The New England Journal of Medicine* divided nearly 8,000 Spanish people who were either overweight or with diabetes into three groups. Each group was given three different diets, including:

a. A Mediterranean diet supplemented with mixed nuts (a mix of hazelnut, walnut or almond).
b. A Mediterranean diet supplemented with extra virgin olive oil.
c. A low-fat diet.

A few scientists examined cardiovascular complications (i.e. heart attack, stroke, death), and the Mediterranean diet. What they noted was that as compared to the control group (with a low-fat diet), the group who followed the Mediterranean diet with high fat (olive oil and nuts) was much less affected by the development of CVD complications. Its risk was reduced by 70 per cent in both intervention groups. These results prove the therapeutic effects of healthy fats on the heart (and overall) health. (27)

Later studies analysing the above data found the addition of high fat to the Mediterranean diet was also associated with a reduction in belly fat, blood pressure, LDL cholesterol, and inflammation. (28,29,30)

A note on virgin coconut oil and butter

Provided that you reduce calories from refined vegetable oil (Omega-6), the nutrients you receive from coconut oil and butter are highly beneficial. Lauric acid, a particular type of medium-chain triglycerides, present in coconut oils helps us to boost metabolism, enhances our brain function and strengthens our immunity. (31)

Traditional Asian cultures (such as India and Thailand) rely on coconut (oil, milk, and cream) for food and even for its anti-fungal and anti-bacterial properties. I grew up in this culture and savoured many delicacies, both sweet and savoury made with coconuts. Ensure that you buy cold-pressed, virgin, organic coconut oil to get its maximum benefits.

Recommended read: 'Eat Fat Get Thin' by Dr Mark Hayman busts many myths about the fallacy of eating a low-fat diet for a healthy life – a great read if you wish to enhance your understanding on this topic.

How you can ensure you enjoy good-quality fat in your eating?

- Remove or limit your intake of vegetable and refined oils.
- Use extra-virgin olive oils or rapeseed oils in your cooking.
- Enjoy small amounts of good-quality coconut oil, grass-fed butter and ghee.

- Enjoy a handful of nuts and seeds as a snack, or nut/seed butter (see recipe below).
- Support your food with a good-quality Omega-3 such as oily fish; or if you are vegetarian, look for vegetarian sources such as flaxseeds or linseeds.
- Use unsweetened nut milk (no preservatives) for your tea and cooking. Making your own is the best option.
- Soak nuts and seeds in water to get the maximum benefit from them and reduce digestive discomfort.
- Enjoy avocado in various forms, salads, guacamoles.

Recipe Suggestions Using Healthy Fats

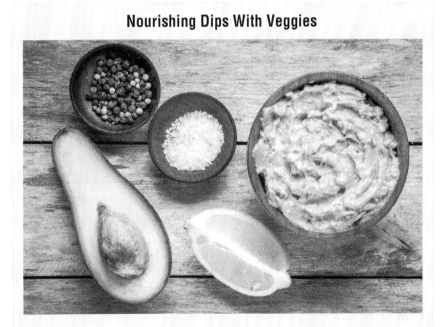

Nourishing Dips With Veggies

This serves as an excellent mid-meal snack. It will give you a feeling of satiety and stop you from overeating at your mealtimes.

Vegetables: choose from following:

- Carrot sticks

- Cucumber sticks
- Sugar-snap peas
- Bell pepper

Dip 1: Nut butter (choose any nuts of your choice like almond, cashew nuts, walnuts or pecans)

- 3 cups raw almonds (soaked overnight and roasted in the oven)
- ¼ teaspoon salt
- Optional: ¼ teaspoon ground cinnamon
- Optional: ½ teaspoon vanilla extract
- Optional: 2 tablespoons maple syrup or honey

Place almonds in a high-speed blender or food processor. Blend until creamy. You may need to pause to scrape down the sides as necessary. You can add remaining ingredients and blend further until it mixes with the almond butter.

Hurray – your nut butter is ready to be savoured!

Dip 2: Guacamole

- 1 ripe avocado, peeled, pitted and chopped
- 2 tsp of lemon juice
- ½ chopped garlic
- Handful of chopped parsley or cilantro
- ¼ cup tomato chopped
- ¼ cup chopped onion
- Pink Himalayan salt and pepper to taste

Place all the ingredients in a mixing jar and pulse the ingredients until well combined. Alternatively, you can also use a fork to create a coarse mixture according to your desired consistency.

Supplements

It is always best to seek all our nutrient requirements from real whole food. However, many people are currently experiencing nutrient deficiencies due to a variety of factors like the quality of soil, levels of chronic stress, and hectic lifestyle. If this is the case, I would encourage you to start this health journey by testing your current nutrients level (by contacting your health provider for testing). Consider taking high-quality supplements to correct any deficiency with the guidance of your health professional.

Supplement recommendations for preventing chronic diseases

(Again, seek professional support before taking them as an excess of external nutrients could cause harm).

- A high-quality multivitamin and mineral or vitamin specific to your deficiencies, like zinc or Vitamin B12
- Vitamin D3
- Probiotics
- Omega-3 (fish oil or vegan source)

Hydration

> *"Water is the driving force of all nature."*
> – Leonardo Da Vinci

Water has been an essential component of many ancient healing modalities. It has been given a status of 'hydrotherapy' offering its therapeutic benefits via hot healing springs across the world. Many interventions in naturopathy science are based on hydrotherapy.

This is no surprise because 70 per cent of our body is made of water. Water is crucial in maintaining our cellular health, energy, and performance. Lack of hydration affects our mood, leads to distress, headache and constipation, and even unhealthy behaviour such as overeating.

How much water to drink?

Thirst is a poor indicator of dehydration. In society today, we drink less water in general. It is especially true when you are experiencing any of the symptoms mentioned above, or your urine is concentrated (aim for pale yellow to clear – this is the standard urine colour).

Follow these **10 hydration strategies** to ensure your body is well hydrated for its optimum performance:

1. Choose your water source carefully if you are living in an area where there is high salt or fluoride content in your drinking water for health reasons. In that case, it is better to invest in a high-quality water filter or consider purchasing drinking water from a good quality source.
2. Drink at least 8–10 glasses of water each day. Increase the intake if the weather is hot and humid, or your physical activity demands have increased.
3. If you are under the weather or unwell, drink more water and fluids such as soups and fresh juices (diluted if needed) to increase your body fluids.
4. Ensure you are NOT drinking packaged drinks and juices which are readily available in the supermarket. They are full of sugar and preservatives – instead, opt for a water bottle.
5. To get into a routine, set an hourly reminder on the phone to drink ½ a glass of water.
6. Tie two activities together: as soon as you get up, drink one glass; any time you are washing your hands, use it as a cue to drink a few sips of water; when sitting in a train/bus/car to return home from work, drink a few more sips.
7. Drink water to overcome excess eating: drink one glass of water 30 minutes before a meal and in the afternoon – when the craving for a snack and coffee kicks in. resist the temptation and instead drink water (with natural flavours such as lemon or fruits added if needed) and see your cravings gradually disappear.

8. If drinking plain water feels boring, try to flavour it with citrus fruits such as lemon, orange, or grapefruit or add herbs such as mint or rosemary. I have found that slightly cooler water tastes better.

9. In general, Ayurvedic science (more on this later) recommends drinking lukewarm water in small quantities during your meals and room temperature water throughout the day.

10. Give thanks and bless the source of the water. Set the intention as you are drinking: "This water (with its healing properties) is purifying and energising my cells."

Emotional Eating

You are now equipped with the principles of eating for a healthy heart. Still, I am aware that we as human beings are complex animals, and our eating behaviour is continually being influenced by many factors that go beyond scientific guidance and knowledge.

Our thoughts, emotions, harmony and disharmony of our relationship with others and time of the day, our ability to control our stress levels, are all positively or negatively impacting our food choices and notably our digestion.

When we feel blue or have stress at work or in life, we seek comforting food that gives an immediate response of pleasure – such as fried chips, crisps, pizza, or sugary snacks. Eating while we are in a negative state, leads to over-eating, digestive issues, and ultimately, a diseased state.

In the past, when eating alone, I made little or no effort in cooking a big meal and often sat in front of the TV/YouTube, not realising the quantity of food I was consuming, even if it was healthy. We all have been there – agree?

While recovering from stress-related digestive issues, I sought an expert Ayurvedic doctor, Dr Sameer Jamdagni, in India. Along with his Ayurvedic interventions and lifestyle recommendations, he encouraged me to calm my mind-body before and while eating. As a result, my digestive symptoms recovered significantly, and so did my emotional eating.

Here, I present the Healthy Eating Principles based on Ayurveda, mindfulness, and emotional wellness. They will assist you to overcome emotional eating and extract maximum nourishment from every bite you are eating.

Healthy Eating Principles to Nourish Mind, Body and Soul:

1. Eat only when you are hungry

A popular belief prevalent in today's society is that we have to eat three meals and two or more snacks. Admittingly, to balance insulin levels, we have to ensure our body gets some supply of food. However, it is unnecessary to consume a massive portion of breakfast when your body is still digesting food from the previous day.

Giving time and space for digestion to occur is crucial, even if it means delaying the time for your first meal of the day, this is fine. Do not let the clock guide your eating behaviour. Respect your body's rhythm, and then decide the times of your meals. For example, if you don't feel hungry until 10am or 11am, but 'social norms' force you to eat breakfast at 8am, stop that habit.

Your physiological needs are different than others in your family. Make a seven-day diary of your hunger response to find out your biorhythms for eating meals and then stick to them.

2. Routine

Ayurveda recommends having a routine for our meals with our main meal in the afternoon between 12 am and 2 pm, when our digestive power is at its highest. Due to work pressure, if this is not always possible, consider having your dinner as early in the day as you can, preferably no later than 7 pm.

3. Mindful eating:

Never eat on autopilot in front of the TV or when you have had an argument. Applying some stress management strategies before a meal can help you. Calm yourself with 5–10 deep breaths or just lying in sav asana (corpse pose) to let yourself settle down before eating in a relaxing environment. A review of RCTs has shown that applying stress management strategies was associated with a reduction in weight and emotional eating behaviour. (32)

Be mindful of your posture while eating. When you sit in a comfortable position rather than stand or slouch, you allow your digestive system to work at its maximum capacity.

Enjoy the eating experience; preferably share this in the company of friends or family. Remember, eating is a social activity rather than mere calorie intake.

Set the intention that **<u>"This meal/drink will nourish my body, mind and spirit."</u>**

Bless the food, cook, and company you are eating with and savour each bite, the texture, taste, aroma of the food, and the pleasant conversation you hear over the table. Let your meal be a multi-sensory experience.

4. What are you hungry for?

In his book, 'What Are You Hungry For?' author, cardiologist and pioneer of mind-body integration medicine, Dr Deepak Chopra offers some of the best advice to overcome emotional eating. Taking inspiration from his teachings, I have created my own version of overcoming emotional eating,

When you find yourself, eating countless servings or your favourite food or snacking even after you finished a hearty meal, take the following steps:

A. Become self-aware that you are leaning towards emotional eating.

Notice your breathing and tension in your body to bring your awareness from out there into your being.

Ask the following questions:

"Am I really hungry? Or am I thirsty?" See if drinking a glass of water would assist you in overcoming the urge to reach for that chocolate.
"How hungry am I?"
"What am I really hungry for?"

From my personal experience and what I hear from my clients, emotional eating is more than about food.

See what applies to you and try to substitute some of these activities instead of stress eating – moments when stress would otherwise lead us to snack.

- **Need for love**: This is the most profound need every human has. When we feel isolated or sad, we lose connection with our bodies and indulge in toxic-eating patterns. Numerous scientific evidences has shown a strong link between lack of social support and interaction with emotional eating. (33,34)

    If this has been your experience, see if you can create more loving experiences by giving and receiving more love in your life. Call your friend or speak to your neighbour or pet your dog or cat, cuddle a child, or express self-love by gifting yourself time for a relaxing bath, a sensuous massage, or even a weekend getaway.

- **Need for fun and stimulation**: Boredom and routine create monotony in our lives; we try to overcome this by eating a variety of foods. Instead, throughout your day or week, you could plan different activities: go for a walk, take up a new hobby such as dance, learn guitar, meet new people, explore other parts of your city. These more unique experiences will stimulate you and will enrich your life in more rewarding ways than eating, (you will achieve a renewed zest for life).

- **Reframe limiting thoughts to positive empowering beliefs**: Our experience creates limiting beliefs in our subconscious that make change harder. As a child, if your parents always forced you to finish the food on your plate, when you become an adult that voice still rings in your ears. If the majority of your family or friends overeat, it is easy to normalise this behaviour. I would encourage you to identify these patterns and thoughts that may be limiting you in your desire to eat healthily. Know that your past is not equal to your future, and with newer knowledge and motivation, you can create positive changes in your eating behaviour.

Reframe your thoughts with these positive, empowering thoughts:

- I am light.
- My body, mind, and spirit are in harmony (while eating).
- I am in control of the food I am consuming.
- I nourish my mind with stimulating thoughts and experiences and meaningful work.
- I feed my soul by sharing love, compassion, and joy.
- I nourish my body with life-giving fresh, living food and drinks.

B. Environmental changes to promote healthy eating and a positive lifestyle

Create following changes in your environment:

1. Enjoy meals in a happy environment, preferably in the company of family and friends.
2. Enjoy a multi-sensory approach: light a candle, put on soothing music, inhale a light scent while eating.
3. Before any meal, bless and thank the food to enhance its healing properties. If you have company, thank them for sharing an important aspect of their life with you.
4. Sattvic cooking: Ever wonder why your mum's food tasted the best you ever had? This is because it's been cooked with the emotion of 'Pure Love.' Food cooked calmly with the feelings of pure love for those who you are cooking for enhances the quality of the food, nourishing mind, body, and soul.

Ayurvedic principles for healthy eating

Ayurveda is an art and science of traditional Indian medicine. The word 'ayu' means life and 'ved' means knowledge in Sanskrit: 'Knowledge of Life'. Ayurveda aims to heal diseases and maintain the person's optimum health; therefore adopting its principles is useful in both the prevention and control of lifestyle-related diseases.

Ayurvedic Constitutes

According to Ayurveda, every human being is formed of 3 different constituents called doshas – namely Vata, Pitta, and Kapha. The following table illustrates these three doshas.

	Vata	Pitta	Kapha
Predominant Element	Space and Air	Fire and Water	Water and Earth
Use/Governs	Movement within the body and emotions.	Digestive system, and body temperature.	Inflammation.
Balance	• Energising movements and joints. • Contentment/ balanced emotion.	• Healthy digestion and elimination. • Equilibrium of temperature / weight.	• Balance weight. • Optimum health.
Imbalance	• Joint pain/stiffness in muscles. • Anxiety/feelings of sadness.	• Digestive-related issues. • Excessive perspiration, inflamed skin, inflammation of the body. • Anger, hate, jealousy.	• Obesity. • Diabetes and other chronic diseases.

Reference: 35

"A lifestyle based on Ayurvedic principles leads to the creation of optimum health and vitality."
—Pranita Salunke

Gunas (Qualities of nature):

Ayurveda divides food and lifestyle according to 3 different qualities: Sattvic, Tamasic, and Rajasic. By enhancing the Sat quality food and lifestyle, this ensures the balance of our constituents and health.

The following table gives essential guidance of lifestyle related to these three qualities.

	Sattvic	**Rajasic**	**Tamasic**
Meaning	Purity	Passion	Impurity
Promotes	The science of Ayurveda promotes the benefit of leading a Sattvic lifestyle to enhance our health. • It brings purity and calmness to the mind. • It enhances spiritual development – helping us to build compassion, ability to forgive, create detachment and ability to love another being at a deeper level.	Promotes actions and drive, hence it is important to have balanced Rajasic to undertake new challenges and achieve goals. An excess of passionate food and lifestyle increases restlessness and overactivity.	Indulging in Tamasic lifestyle creates a lack of lustre and vigour in one's mind leading to laziness, lack of motivation and lack of purpose in life. This lifestyle also produces many mental and physical health conditions.
Food	Vital food: Food with Prana which means life-force. Natural food, which is pure, whole and naturally delicious.	Animal products. Spices Foods and drinks with extreme tastes of: spicy, salty, bitter, pungent, dry, hot.	Frozen, packaged canned and processed food. Stale food. Caffeinated food and drinks.

	Sattvic	Rajasic	Tamasic
¬	Fresh, vibrant colour; seasonal fruits and vegetables. Wholesome grains, nuts and seeds. Sprouts. Freshly prepared food. • Eating according to seasonal variations. In winter: (Vata season) * Eating warm and grounding foods such as wholesome grains and soups nourished with healthy fats such as olive oil, butter/ghee or avocados. In Spring: (kaph season) The body is prone to lung infection, therefore food to dry mucous from the body such as greens, honey, grains like millet. Summer (Pitta season): meals which have cooling properties: juices, salads, light fruits and vegetables. Ayurveda also emphasises the importance of *Mitahara* – literally meaning the habit of eating moderate food.		Indulgence in alcohol, drugs.
Sleep	Sound sleep according to the biological cycle, between 10 pm–5 am.	Light sleep	Erratic sleep schedule
Thought patterns	Driven by emotions of non-violence, surrender, appreciation, kindness, compassion, love, joy, contentment.	Arrogance, ego, uncontrollable desires, fear, jealousy, hate, anger, overthinking.	Feelings of sadness, apathy, loss of direction, depression, ignorance, lethargy.

	Sattvic	Rajasic	Tamasic
Health	Sattvic lifestyle and food are nourishing, healing, and energising. Easy to digest.	Excessive Rajasic lifestyle leads to anxiety, stress, self-centeredness and insomnia	Indulging in Tamasic lifestyle leads to development of chronic diseases and therefore premature death. Impact of Tamasic lifestyle goes beyond life years. It damages the quality of our thoughts; we lose the ability to be productive and lead an enriching, successful life.

Reference: 35, 36

"Leading a Sattvic lifestyle means: enjoying high-quality live food in our diet, with a balance of tastes, and eliminating processed, dead food; moving joyfully, thinking positively, cultivating pure virtues and working according to our innate purpose leads to a healthy and happy heart."
—Pranita Salunke

CHAPTER 7

Joyful Movement

"If you want your heart to be healthy, mind to be strong and spirit to be alive, then you need to move more. It's that simple."
—Pranita Salunke

When we are engaged in any physical activity, billions of cells in our body are interacting with the environment and forming new neuronal pathways. This enhances our health, happiness, creativity, work performance, self-image and confidence.

Wouldn't it be nice if we could find immense joy in moving throughout our day and making it a part of our life as opposed to making it as a chore that we are forced to do?

"You have been given one stomach to eat consciously and two legs to move DAILY and not just a few times a week."
—Pranita Salunke

By enjoying any physical activities – like walking in the park, along the seashore, dancing to your favourite tunes, lifting weights, or playing football in the field – we are working on a vital lifestyle element that will keep our heart healthy and happy, a great gift we can give to ourselves.

Benefits of active lifestyle

The World Health Organisation warns us about the dangers of a sedentary lifestyle. Physical inactivity is ranked as the fourth largest risk factor for dying early and it contributes to the development of heart diseases.

On a positive note, for all of us, including those with a high risk of chronic diseases, an improvement in your aerobic capacity or fitness level even by one unit will lessen the chances of early uncalled-for death by 8–17%.(1) An improvement in physical fitness is determined by Metabolic Equivalent (MET). 1 MET= 3.5 ml/O2/kg/min. The fitness level of above 7 METs has been associated with the lowest CVD risk.(2) People with already established heart disease also benefit from regular physical activity. A meta-analysis [5] of RCTs demonstrated a 20% reduction in death due to all causes and a 26% reduction in dying from heart conditions.(3)

According to a study published in the *Heart* international cardiology journal, researchers observed 57,000 people with a median age of 53. Participants performed treadmill stress tests, which test exercise capacity. The study then followed them for ~ ten years for all-cause mortality and ~5 years for myocardial infarction (heart attack). The study found that each improvement in MET (exercise capacity) was associated with an 18% reduction in risk of death in those under 40 and a 12% reduction in those over 70.(4)

You don't necessarily have to know the science behind calculating exercise capacity to enjoy the benefits of exercise. Just know that moving more is better for your heart, mind and soul.

Some of the benefits of physical activities:

- Exercise and physical and mental health: joyfully moving can calm many of the symptoms of depression, such as fatigue, tension, anger, and reduced vigour.
- Stress plays a significant factor in heart attacks and other physical conditions: exercise is a great stress management tool as it decreases stress hormones like cortisol in our body.

---

[5] A meta-analysis: an examination of data from a number of independent studies of the same subject in order to determine an overall trend.

- Joyfully moving increases 'feel-good' hormones like endorphins and serotonin, giving your mood a natural boost. This brings a sense of calm and peace.
- Exercise takes your focus away from the problems of your life and creates mindfulness as you focus on the activity you are enjoying and also assists in increasing your resilience.
- Group sports like football, cricket, rugby or trekking in a group are social activities; you can enjoy the benefit of social support which is very important for mental wellness.
- Various activities and exercise help you to lower your risk of cardiovascular disease and help prevent many other chronic diseases like diabetes, hypertension and even cancer.
- Exercise improves your metabolism and your body's use of insulin. Therefore, it assists in normalising weight and blood sugar control.

8 Principles for Healthier and Happier Physical Activities

1. Before you start to exercise, it is always best to get a green signal from your doctor – especially if you are suffering from any health conditions or pain. Your health practitioner is aware of your medical history and current medications, which can all play a role in your ability to exercise.

2. Other lifestyle factors must be in place before you undertake any intense exercise plan to ensure your exercises are building your physique rather than causing damage. Ensure you are sleeping optimally and eating nourishing food before sweating intensely in the gym or outside. If you must join a 6am spin class, go to bed early at night, and prepare your meals for the coming week.

3. Choose activities that are fun and more meaningful to you to keep you motivated and to make sure the new habits are sustainable.

When I joined a new health club, in my initial excitement I joined many classes including body pump with weights and spin. With both activities, I had very little interest and I felt exhausted and continuously hungry, only to give up after a few sessions.

I realised that if I stuck to my favourite forms of movement, then my fitness journey would be much more enjoyable. For me, they were:

- Yoga: that stretches my mind and body; building strength by using my body weight (calisthenic) and holding the poses while breathing consciously enhances my body awareness and balance.
- Dancing (especially to the tunes of Bollywood): it's a great form of exercise for endurance, balance and coordination.
- Walking/running in nature: increasing my heart health and getting vitamin D from nature giving me double benefits.
- Swimming: this is an excellent exercise for my heart, toning my arms and legs and also calming the mind.

Exercise:

What are your favourite forms of exercise that stimulate and strengthen your body and mind?

Yoga
Tai Chi
Aerobic Exercise
Running
Dance
Weightlifting
Any others?

4. Make physical activity a social event filled with fun. Join a group class, exercise or walk with your family/partner.

   Play a sport with your kids.

Put on inspirational music when you move.

5. Progressive overload: start your exercise with less intensity and for a shorter duration and gradually build up as you listen to your body and adjust to give your body a chance to recover.

6. No pain, no gain! How many of us fall prey of this myth: you have to push through the pain to gain muscle mass and improve fitness?

    Apart from some muscle soreness within 24 to 48 hours of engaging in (new/strenuous) exercise, science terms it as of DOMS (delayed onset muscle soreness), all pain factors must be carefully addressed. Some of the common complaints my clients present with, especially before engaging in any exercise plan are, low back and neck pain due to long hours of sitting at the computer, and shoulder pain due to driving for long hours or carrying heavy work bags. These pain issues can be addressed by manipulation techniques such as osteopathy, physiotherapy or massage therapies.

    My advice is: always manage your pain before starting any activity and exercise plan.

7. Posture: it is important to focus on optimum biomechanical alignment and correct posture to get the maximum benefit from your exercise and activities. You may have noted differences in misalignment in postures while people are using weights at the gym. In the long-term, this has detrimental effects on joints and soft tissues and makes you susceptible to joint pain or injuries.

    As an Occupational Therapist, before advising any physical activities or exercise, I complete biomechanical and posture assessment. If any issues are noted, then clients are advised to correct the misalignment with specific therapies or movements.

    My advice for you is to look in the mirror and observe the alignment of your shoulder, hips, knees and feet while standing, sitting and walking. If you are having any trouble, a visit to a physiotherapist or osteopath will better prepare you for an active life ahead.

8. Variety is the key! Rather than focusing on one type of exercise, choose a combination of activities that you enjoy, and this gives you the benefit of improving all aspects of fitness such as endurance, strength, flexibility, balance, coordination and agility.

My intention in this book is to inspire you to look at physical activities as a part of your life and choose the activity programme that gives YOU the most joy. For me, it is yoga, so let's discuss a few yogic poses to improve overall fitness and health. The scope of the book is to inspire you towards your chosen activities and is not meant to give an in-depth exercise plan. There are many instructional videos available on the web to suit different styles. Choose the ones you gravitate towards. Above all, have fun in your movement and enjoy the process of exploration.

Yoga offers benefits in improving the majority of fitness components as well as its own health benefits.

Studies published in *Complementary Therapies in Clinical Practice* found that yoga can help with the following: (5,6,7)

- Improves quality of life.
- Lowers heart rate.
- Lowers blood pressure.
- Improves respiration.
- Reduces the stress response.
- Reduces depression and anxiety.
- Increases energy and feelings of well-being.

Best Yoga and Pranayama Timings

To get its full benefit, the best time to perform yoga and pranayama is in the early morning, with a fresh breeze and sunrise. Some of the restorative poses and breathing can also be practised in the evening.

During the mid-day slump: if you feel sluggish a few hours after lunch, enjoy these techniques to immediately increase your energy rather than reaching for a coffee or cookie.

Precautions:

Before starting any new programme, including yoga and pranayama, it is always best to seek medical advice and to do these exercises under supervision.

If you are suffering from any chronic conditions or heart disease, it is vital that you perform it under the supervision of an experienced instructor. (The information presented here is for education purposes only – it is not a substitute for professional medical advice, diagnosis, or treatment)

7 Yogic Poses To Enhance Health And Happiness

1. Empowering breath

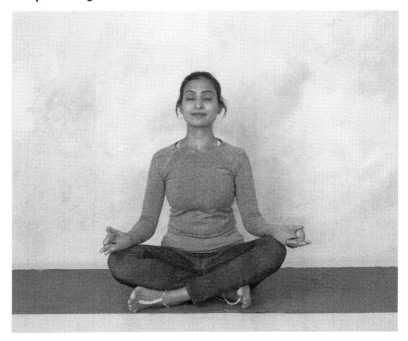

Use this breath to receive inspiration and centre your body and mind.

- Sit in a comfortable position, with an extended spine.
- Breathe in pure air and breathe out impurity of thoughts.
- Breathe in vitality and breathe out lethargy.
- Breathe in focus and breathe out confusion.
- Breathe in health and breathe out disease.
- Breathe in joy and breathe out pain.

Visualise energy gently moving from the base of your spine to the top of your head as you focus on your breath. Bring awareness to your mind and ask for inspiration from your higher self – an inspiration to be a better version of yourself. Practise this breathing in each of the following poses, focusing on breathing through the energetic channel along your spine.

2. Chair Pose (Utkatasana)

Chair Pose stimulates the function of the diaphragm and heart and strengthens arms, legs and core. Strengthening our heart helps us acknowledge our connection to all things. We can breathe and move into the future with more power and conviction.

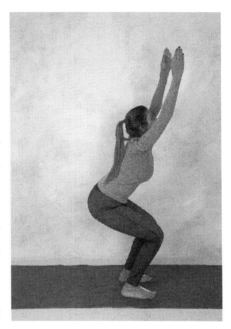

- From standing position, inhale and raise your arms.
- Exhale and bend your knees until they are parallel to the floor, ensuring your knees do not cross your toes.
- Maintain that clear line of energy along your spine by engaging your abdominal muscles.
- Keep the spine elongated by engaging your shoulders and moving your tailbone towards the ground.
- Open your chest by lifting strongly through the arms.
- As you find the sweet spot of strength and balance between front and back, future and past, stay here for five conscious breaths, then release your arms as you come to a standing position.

Contraindications and Cautions

- Headache
- Insomnia
- Low blood pressure

3. Half Lord of the Fishes Pose

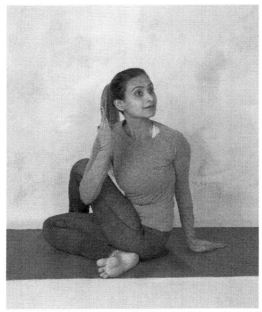

Ardha Matsyendra-asana (Ardha = half Matsyendra = king of the fish)

This pose stimulates your internal organs, kidney, liver, pancreas and is immensely helpful for digestive disorders, weight issues and diabetes control. The pose also helps to awaken our serpent energy, called Kundalini.

- From a long sitting position bring the sole of your right foot close to your left hip by bending your right knee.
- Inhale to lengthen your spine; exhale to twist towards the right side of your body.
- Be mindful of the twist in your spine as you lengthen your torso, and firmly keep both buttocks on the ground.
- Stay here for five conscious breaths, lengthening and twisting with each inhalation and trying to relax with each exhalation.

Contraindications and Cautions

- Back or spine injury.

4. Revolved Side Angle Pose (Parivrtta Parsvakonasana)

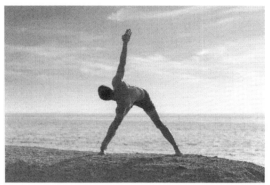

Extended Triangle Pose (Utthita Trikonasana)

Extended Triangle Pose is a posture that helps you stay grounded while connecting to the unbounded universe. It improves circulation in your lower spine and internal organs, including the abdomen and pelvic organs. It improves balance and enhances your strength.

- From standing pose (tadasana), step your legs 2–3 feet apart; turn your right foot out 90 degrees and your left foot in slightly.
- As you breathe in, extend your arms out to your sides.
- Breathe out and reach outside of the right foot.
- Be mindful of stabilising your pelvis and lengthening your spine before placing your right hand on the floor or a block under your right shoulder.
- Your left hand reaches to the sky while maintaining a beautiful alignment of both the arms.
- Stay in this pose for five deep breaths as you observe your breath energising your spine and internal organs. Inhale and come up, pivot your feet, as you practise the pose on the other side before returning to Tadasana (Mountain Pose).

Contraindications and Cautions

- Headache
- High or low blood pressure
- Insomnia

5. Bow Pose (Dhanurasana):

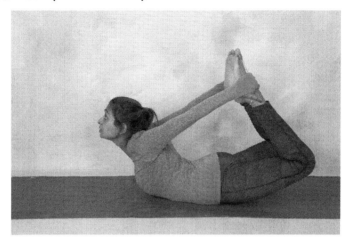

This is a back-strengthening pose that opens your shoulders and chest and on an energetic level works on unblocking your heart chakra – a site for the expression of love and connection.

This pose is also beneficial to improve hip flexibility and energising all internal organs and digestion.

- From a prone position, bend your knees, and reach for your feet or ankles.
- As you inhale, lift your torso and head and press your feet up toward the sky, helping you to lift your chest higher.
- Activate the strength of your leg muscles, stabilise your pelvis as you gently bend your spine and open your heart, and gaze towards the sky.
- Hold here for five deep breaths and then slowly release to the floor. Repeat up to 3 times.

Contraindications and Cautions

- High or low blood pressure
- Migraine
- Insomnia
- Serious lower back or neck injury

6. Warrior II Pose:

For a fierce warrior inside you, an incarnation of Lord Shiva, this Warrior Pose increases your overall body strength and sharpens your focus so that you can achieve success in your goals.

- From the Mountain Pose, step your feet approximately 4 feet apart. Turn your right foot to the right and your left foot out to the left 90 degrees, as you raise your arms parallel to the floor with palms down.
- Bend your right knee to a 90-degree angle while maintaining the alignment with right and left feet.
- As you take five conscious breaths, reach out your arms actively on both sides with feet firmly on the ground. Now, turn your eyes (focus) to the right side of your body and visualise attainment of your goals with the strength you are receiving from this warrior practice.
- Inhale and come up, pivot your feet, as you practise the pose on the other side before returning to Tadasana.

Contraindications and Cautions

- Diarrhoea
- High blood pressure
- Neck problems: don't turn your head to look over your front hand; continue to look straight ahead with both sides of your neck lengthened evenly.

7. Corpse Pose (Savasana):

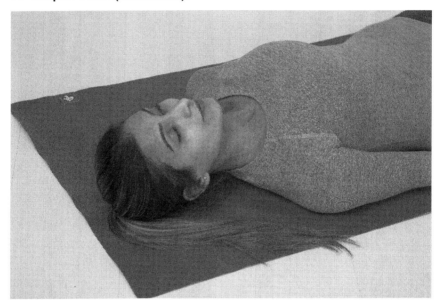

Surrender your mind to the universe as you totally relax your body. Lie on your back, with your spine in a neutral position. If you have a lower back issue, support your legs with a few cushions. Keep your palms facing the sky and close your eyes. Notice the thoughts that drift through your head, thoughts of where you think you should be or what you should be doing; let them pass like clouds in the sky. Keep your awareness to the present moment of deep relaxation and pure joy. Stay in this pose for as long as you wish to enjoy the experience.

Prana-Yam

"Feelings come and go like clouds in a windy sky.
Conscious breathing is my anchor."
—Thich Nhat Hanh

Prana is a vital force that pulsates through every human being giving us life and energy. Prana is a Sanskrit term for a breath. We experience fatigue, lethargy, reduced vigour and even health issues as a result of improper breathing or Prana. The regular practice of conscious breathing patterns called pranayama (extension of breath) will not only improve your lung function, but it will also restore your vigour, vital force, our Prana. Pranayama is different from our usual breathing which is regulated automatically and unconsciously.

By cultivating more 'Prana', we will enjoy enhanced mental clarity, peace and strong connection with self, energising all our activities and interactions with others. Imagine how your life-experience would be enhanced if you could increase your vitality 10%–20%–50%–100%? You would be invincible and able to achieve all your goals and dreams and enjoy life with its full glory.

Pranayama Improves Cardiovascular Health

Various studies have shown that pranayama practice is beneficial for cardiovascular functions because it is useful for dealing with the effects of stress, and it normalises blood pressure levels. A study carried out by the Departments of Physiology and Advanced Centre for Yoga Therapy, Education & Research, in Pondicherry, examined that when participants underwent slow pranayama training for 30 minutes, three times a week for the duration of 12 weeks, they experienced significant improvements in the levels of perceived stress, heart rate, respiratory rate, systolic blood pressure and diastolic blood pressure. (8) Increasing evidence from scientific researchers clearly demonstrates that yoga and pranayama together can decrease levels of salivary cortisol and blood glucose, offering protection against metabolic conditions, including insulin resistance and type 2 diabetes.(9)

Here, I share two Pranayama practices which have helped my clients and me to improve overall health and wellness:

1. Bhastrika: Deep-Diaphragmatic Breathing

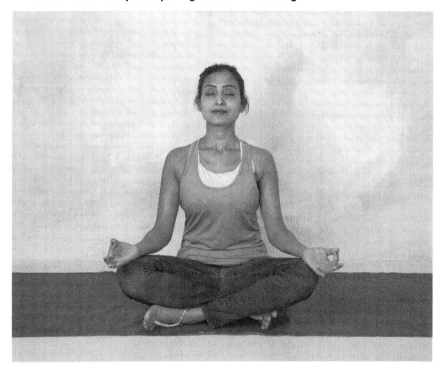

Bhastrika or "bellows breath," is an effective breathing technique that helps to increase Prana or life force in your body. The Sanskrit word "Bhastrika" means "bellows" (such as those used by blacksmiths when melting metal). Similar to the bellows' action in fanning the fire, Bhastrika Pranayama infuses the flow of air into the body to increase the energetic force at both the physical and subtle level – the inner fire of mind and body.

Benefits:

- Removes lethargy and laziness by energising your body and mind.
- This pranayama improves digestion capacity, boosts your metabolism and helps you to lose weight.
- Strengthens and tones the abdominal region.
- Calms the mind.
- Oxygenates the blood, increasing the vitality of all the organs and tissues.
- Improves lung function.

How to Perform Bellows Breath:

1. Sit up tall, relax your shoulders and close your eyes.
2. Take deep breaths in from your nose and expand your belly fully as you breathe; your diaphragm descends as your lungs expand.
3. Now, exhale forcefully through your nose.
4. Inhale and exhale repeatedly, deeply and forcefully.
5. Make sure you are not breathing from your mouth, your body is aligned, and your breath is coming from your diaphragm.
6. There will be a strong nasal sound accompanying this breathing and breathing is rhythmic and controlled, maintaining the speed as per your capacity.
7. Do ten rounds of Bhastrika breaths. Momentarily pause while breathing naturally and repeat for three times.
8. Always listen to your body: if you experience any discomfort, or feel light-headed, pause, let it pass and then practise it slowly.

Contraindications:

Do not practise Bhastrika if you're pregnant, have uncontrolled hypertension, epilepsy, seizures, or panic disorder.

You should also avoid practising bellows breath on a full stomach; wait at least two hours after eating. Practise under supervision of a practitioner if you are suffering from heart ailments, high blood pressure, fever, vertigo, pregnancy, intestinal disorders, spinal abnormalities and eye ailments, (e.g. detached retina, glaucoma.)

Avoid practising bellows breathing close to sleep time, as it may invigorate your mind and make it difficult to fall asleep.

2. "Alternate nostril breathing" (in Sanskrit, this is called Anulom-Vilom or Nadi Shodhana).

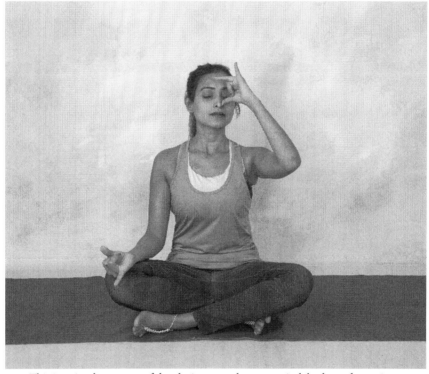

This is a simple yet powerful technique to calm your mind, body, and emotions.

Benefits of Alternate Nostril Breathing

- Alternate nostril breaths will help you to calm your nerves and ease your thoughts when you are experiencing a stressful situation, (such as a job interview, an important meeting, public speaking, dealing with conflict at work, etc.)

- Aligns your energy and restores inner balance when you are overthinking, feeling anxious or stressed.
- If done before meditation, you will enjoy more benefit from your practice as it immediately brings more clarity to your mind.
- Restores balance in the left and right sides of the brain. The left side of the brain is governed by logic, step-by-step processes, practical aspects of life; masculine energy which is important for the completion of the tasks. When this is balanced by the power of the right side of the brain (which is a site of intuition, creativity, ideas, flow state) then you can really savour joy and harmony in life.
- Regular practise of this powerful technique opens up the subtle Pranic (Vital) energetic channel.
- According to Ayurvedic science, our body is governed by three doshas and Tridoshas (three doshas) namely Vata, Pitta and Kapha. Regular practice of Anulom-Vilom pranayama helps to balance all three doshas.
- It enhances our physical energy by improving functions of the lungs and nervous system and removing toxins. It therefore benefits respiratory issues (like asthma and allergies, headaches, snoring) and helps patients with nervous system defects (like paralysis or Parkinson's), where there is an imbalance in muscle groups that would get a huge benefit from its practice.
- It is effective in controlling blood pressure, therefore benefits your heart health.
- Overall health and positivity are enhanced.

How to do Anulom Vilom?

1. Seat yourself comfortably on the mat or in the chair, with a straight spine and an open heart.
2. Close your eyes, or slightly open them to keep your head straight. In this pranayama, the position of your head is key, as it will affect which subtle channel in your spine the energy will flow towards.

3.   Start with both hands placed on your lap, left hand in Gyan mudra, right hand in Vishnu Mudra

Gyan Mudra:

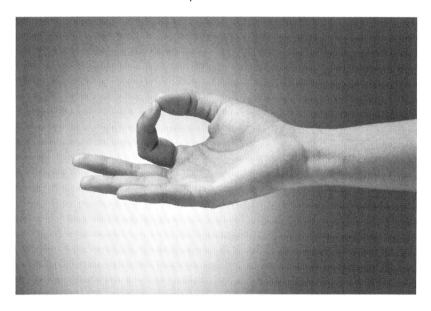

Vishnu Mudra:

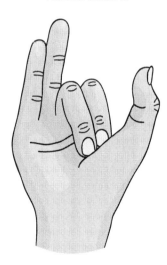

Vishnu Mudra

4. Now close your right nostril with your right thumb and start inhaling slowly from your left nostril and take breaths as much as possible, filling your lungs completely with pure, oxygenated air.

5. Now block both nostrils and hold your breath for 3–4 seconds. (People with health conditions such as cardiac issues or blood pressure patients and pregnant women should not hold their breath while doing this pranayama, just keep inhaling and exhaling.)

6. Now exhale from your right nostril while closing your left nostril with the middle finger.

7. Start repeating this again, this time inhaling from the right nostril; close the left nostril with your middle finger. Now, block both nostrils and hold the breath for 3–4 seconds. Then, exhale from your left nostril while closing your right nostril with the middle finger.

8. This is one cycle: you will do 5 cycles in total.

9. Repeat a maximum of 5–10 cycles, allowing your mind to follow your inhales and exhales.

10. You could change hands to ease the process.

11. During the practice, focus your attention to your breath on the present moment, and if your attention drifts away gently bring your awareness back to the current moment.

CHAPTER 8

Sleep

"Sleep is a nature's gift to start life again, bringing the hope of a new day and the potential for a better future."
—Pranita Salunke

Rejuvenating sleep is one of the foundations for good health. All worries, pressures and pains of the day halt during our restful slumber, rejuvenating our bodies and minds and enhancing our happiness.

Science affirms the importance of sleep in retaining memory, learning new information and maintaining health. Sound sleep repairs our tissues and muscles, and in addition strengthens bones and our immune system. As a baby, our parents ensured that we had a good environment and routine for restful sleep, knowing its importance for our growth.

As we grow, personal and work commitments take priority over this very important aspect of our health. Lack of quality and quantity of sleep leads to a number of serious health troubles, including hormonal disruption, high blood pressure, irregular hunger, obesity and mood disorders. Sleep troubles compromise our length and quality of life by creating many lifestyle-related diseases.

If you have been ignoring good quality sleep, I encourage you to pause and reflect how your current health relates to this important lifestyle element: sleep.

Sleep Awareness Questionnaire:

I am reaffirming that awareness is the key to making positive changes. Complete the following questionnaire for the next seven days and work on the recommendations mentioned here in order to improve the quality and quantity of your sleep. If you notice any sleep-related problems, please visit your primary physician for appropriate interventions.

(Remember: some of the sleep problems could cause a potential threat to your health. However, the harmful effect on your health can be prevented with the right support.)

Sleep Awareness Questionnaire

1. Quantity:

   How many hours of sleep do you get in a 24-hour period?

2. Quality:

   a. Do you have undisturbed sleep?
   b. Do you feel refreshed after waking up?
   c. Do you have difficulty falling asleep or staying asleep?
   d. Do you suffer from inability to focus during the day?
   e. Do you feel a need to sleep during the day excessively?

3. Sleep-related issues:

   a. Do you find yourself tired or unintentionally sleeping during the day, for example, at an important meeting? Or while driving?
   b. Has anyone observed that you stopped breathing while sleeping? (observed apnoea)
   c. Do you suffer from any of the following: snoring, restless leg syndrome or any other issue? (These symptoms affect your ability to maintain adequate restorative sleep).

Adapted from: official publication of the American Academy of Sleep Medicine (1)

The Science Behind Sleep

Let us understand a brief science about how the quality of your sleep is directly related to your health and happiness.

Stages of sleep:

Typically, we pass through the following stages of sleep. We are awake, then we get ready to sleep, and slowly we fall into a light sleep. Gradually, our mind drifts into a deep sleep, (also known as N3, slow-wave or delta-wave sleep) as shown in electroencephalography (EEG).

The majority of our deep sleep occurs during the first half of the night. Effective deep sleep has a restorative function; a better quality of deep sleep means you would feel rested and more alert the next day. This sleep also correlates with the production of growth hormones – therefore, helping you to recover from any injuries or tissue damage, strengthening bones, helping you to look and feel youthful, and improving immunity so that you are less likely to fall sick and you recover well after infection.

Rapid Eye Movement, REM sleep (which is also called a dream sleep), is followed by a cycle of light and deep sleep. Science links the benefits of REM sleep to memory processing and brain functioning such as concentration and improved attention span. Disturbance in REM sleep is also associated with mood problems and even depression.

Why Does Sleep Get Disrupted?

Our society is suffering from sleep deprivation. According to a scientific review published by The National Institute for Health between 50 million and 70 million people do not get enough sleep.(2) Knowing the importance of sleep to our health and wellness, why do we as a global society suffer from chronic sleep deprivation?

Many factors can contribute to the disruption of our sleep:

- Our mood (constant worry or being sad).
- Our lifestyle choices and health issues.

- Work pressure (inability to quieten racing thoughts about upcoming projects).
- Work schedules (long hours, shift-work, etc.)
- Environmental influences, including major life events or habits of our sleeping partner.

Due to any of these situations, we may experience difficulty in sleeping or waking up early or frequently throughout the night. Irrespective of the reason for the sleep problems, we miss on the healing power of sleep.

Sleep and health

Science has shown strong influences of poor-quality sleep on our health.

Eating Habits and Obesity:

Observation of more than 83,377 adults by a public health researcher found that sleeping less than 7 hours increases the risk of obesity by up to 40%. (3)

In the Nurses' Health Study, researchers observed nearly 60,000 women for sixteen years on various aspects of lifestyle. Analysis of the study found that women who slept 5 hours or less per night had a 15% per cent higher risk of obesity than those who slept seven or more hours per night.(4)

How does lack of sleep contribute and lead to obesity, diabetes and heart diseases?

- Lack of sleep disrupts the balance of key hormones that control appetite, gherin and leptin. Gherin triggers the hunger response, and leptin is associated with satiety. Science has shown that people who sleep less have increased gherin and reduced leptin levels. This may contribute to overeating (even of healthier food) and reaching for unhealthy sweet and savoury snacks throughout the day as our impulse control ability is reduced as well.
- Less energy due to poor sleep means less motivation to exercise and be active.

I have certainly experienced this unhealthy behaviour when I don't sleep well. Does this resonate with you?

- Another reason could be that people who don't get enough sleep are awake more, therefore, have more time and opportunity to eat.

Sleep, heart health and diabetes

The unhealthy responses to poor quality of sleep often impair your insulin control and the body's inflammation. *Harvard Heart Letter* warns that sleep deprivation not only increases the risk of developing type 2 diabetes but can take you to an early grave by creating higher blood levels of stress hormones leading to chronic inflammation, which contributes in developing heart diseases including heart attack. (5) In addition, a scientific study published in the *Journal of Sleep Research* found a strong relationship between sleep disturbance and deprivation with an increase in the risk of developing type 2 diabetes and the route to an early grave with heart diseases including heart attack. (6)

Numerous scientists agree that in order to effectively prevent and control the risk of cardiovascular diseases and lifestyle conditions, we have to effectively manage our quality and quantity of sleep. (7)

Sleep Apnoea

Sleep apnoea is a sleep disorder that occurs when your breathing repeatedly stops and starts throughout the night. Sleep apnoea is a well-characterised risk factor for cardiometabolic diseases, including diabetes, and also increases the chances of dying from cardiovascular diseases. Researchers in a study published in *Diabetes Care* found that 86% of participants had sleep apnoea in addition to suffering from diabetes. (8)

Sleep and Mental Health

Prolonged sleep deprivation and insomnia are linked with the development of serious psychological conditions, including depression and bipolar disorders. (9, 10)

Have you noticed how wonderful you feel after a good night's sleep? When your sleep is broken, or you don't get sufficient sleep, you get easily upset or may feel a bit down? I have been there myself on dozens of occasions and let me tell you, my son is not happy to be around me when I wake up after just a few hours of sleep.

I encourage you to view sleep as an important element of your lifestyle, a natural gift to restore your health and physiology, bringing you happiness and hope for a better tomorrow. I hope you are now determined to optimise and enjoy your sleep.

Let us look at some of the ways we can enhance the quality and quantity of our sleep.

1. How much sleep is enough?

When it comes to the 'quantity' of sleep, listen to your body:

There is a great debate on how much sleep is essential, as various researchers are giving different numbers on the adequate amount of sleep. The requirement for sleep varies according to age; babies need more sleep than adults as their brain, physiological and psychological functions are developing.

Also, during illness and stressful periods of our life, we would benefit from more hours of quality sleep to assist in effective healing and recovery.

During our lifestyle assessment, one client reported to me, (with a sense of accomplishment in his tone): "I can perform effectively even with 5 hours of sleep. I have been doing this for the last 20 years, and I feel refreshed after waking up. So why do I need to focus on increasing the quantity of my sleep?"

My response: "If your body is completely disease-free, you are happy with your weight and energy at the end of the day and no other areas of your life are being affected with your current sleep hours, then continue it.

However, if you wish to improve any areas of your physical and mental health, we need to address this core lifestyle behaviour."

Exercise: Complete a sleep diary (as mentioned earlier) and observe the hours of sleep with your mood, energy levels and appetite on that day.

2. **Sleep Environment**: Having an environment that ensures good quality sleep is important. Here are a few suggestions to create a good environment.

- Avoid bright and blue lights in the evening. Blue light emitted from the screens of your TV/computer reduce the body's natural production of melatonin, a substance that plays a role in sleep and other body functions such as hormonal regulation and immune function. Constant Wi-Fi signals are dangerous to your health and the quality of your sleep. Consider having a rule in your household, that all electronic devices, including TV, are not to enter the bedroom. It will not only enhance the quality of your sleep but also your communication with your partner.

  If you must use screens occasionally, consider using screen dimmer apps (e.g. software like flux), or turn on the night and aeroplane mode of your smartphone.

- Human beings sleep better in a dark and quieter space; consider switching to dark curtains or use an eye mask.

- Invest in a comfortable mattress, beautiful bed linens and make your bed as soon as you wake up so that it will welcome you at night for restorative sleep.

- Turn off the notifications from emails and social media that distract you throughout your day from your focus on health, wellness and success in your life.

- If, like me, you are a 'light sleeper' you may like to invest in a good quality earplug to block any noise. Alternatively, you could also have a 'white noise' such as calming music or a fan in the background while you drift off to sleep, so that sudden noise, will not interrupt your sleep. Any low-frequency continuous sound can be used as white noise – as simple as having a fan in your room or installing the latest white noise gadget that plays melodies such as ocean waves to soothe you to sleep.

- Environmental cues: you may have seen young kids sleep so comfortably with their favourite toys. One of the reasons is that this gives them a sense of familiarity and comfort. Hence, I would encourage you to keep one consistent environment cue at hand – both at home or travelling outside – so that like a little child, you can find comfort and familiarity for restorative sleep.

Suggestions: favourite pillow / lavender oil /comfortable woollen blanket throw you can associate with comfort and restful slumber.

3. Health behaviours for optimum sleep: Adopting these healthy habits will ensure that you wake up without the need of your alarm, feeling refreshed, energized, and ready for an amazing day.

i. The circadian rhythm:

According to the Ayurvedic principle, balancing the circadian rhythm of day and night with our body and having regular sleeping and wake-up times harmonises our sleep cycle and health. Early waking to welcome sunrise is encouraged in many traditional Asian cultures. Follow the circadian rhythm of light and dark and do not vary too much from day to day.

ii. Movement: Move more, especially outside to get some necessary Vitamin D; this will make your body physically tired. Going for a daily morning walk or a jog in the sunshine signals the start of the day and enhances feel-good serotonin in your body.

iii. Meals: Finish dinner 2–3 hours before bedtime. Avoid heavy, oily and spicy meals at night that create discomfort in your sleep. Have consistent timings for your meals.

iv. Drinks: Keep caffeinated drinks such as tea or coffee to a maximum of 1–2 a day and consume before 3pm so that your body has a chance to get rid of caffeine when the time comes for sleep.

Remember, caffeine's half-life is 7.5 hours, so if you had a tea/coffee at 4pm, you still have half the amount of caffeine in your bloodstream at 11pm.

Instead of a caffeinated drink, opt for fresh herbal teas like fresh ginger, lemon, cinnamon, camomile.

Many sources of caffeine include tea (white, green, black, and oolong), decaffeinated coffee, colas, some non-cola sodas, chocolate, energy drinks, guarana, and yerba mate.

v. A relaxed body and mind ensures a good quality of sleep

Body

Being in any physical discomfort, stiffness, or pain disturbs the quality of our sleep. If you are experiencing any symptoms, you could try the following techniques to relax your body before sleep.

- Regular (professional or self) massage and a warm bath with essential oils like lavender and sandalwood will relax your body and senses. If you have access to sauna rooms, do enjoy regular visits as the warmth of the experience will increase blood flow and release muscle tension, ensuring a good quality sleep.
- Practise yogic poses such as the child pose and headstand. These calming relaxing poses enhance blood supply to your brain, calm your mind and prepare your body for a relaxing and rejuvenating sleep.

Mind

Often, people who are driven have a lot of ideas as they are retiring for bed, which makes it difficult for them to enter into the beautiful world of rest and restoration. Sometimes, an argument with a spouse/family generates anger and makes it difficult for us to relax; sometimes we may suffer from performance anxiety before a big presentation or an important meeting the next day and stay awake for the entire night risking our productivity and, of course, health. If any of these situations apply to you, the following techniques may help you to reduce anxiety, calm your mind and prepare you for a good night's rest.

a. Stream-of-consciousness writing

This technique of stream-of-consciousness writing, I learnt from Julia Cameron, the author of 'Morning Pages' (after I attended a lecture with her publisher Hay House); this technique has helped many successful artists and professionals to free their mind from the past and make space to create more ideas and power for the future. I recommend doing this at night if overthinking is keeping you awake.

As you do this exercise, you may note profound wisdom, learnings or just negative voices in your head – for which you can lovingly respond: "Thank you for sharing this, but I choose to be better, I choose to be positive."

Write in longhand ideas, suggestions, thoughts from your stream of consciousness, any thoughts, or minor niggles that are disturbing you. If racing thoughts are making it difficult for you to relax, write free-hand in your journal and express anything you wish: anger, frustration, worry, sadness. Write until you feel its cathartic effect. Write down exactly how you feel. Once you empty your thoughts on the paper, you will notice the difference in the clarity of your mind.

You can then write three steps you can take in the next few days that are in your control to overcome your worry. Set a timeline: this way, you are putting your brain at rest, knowing you have a plan to overcome obstacles.

b. Progressive muscle relaxation

The intention for this exercise is to notice and relax any tension in your body, calm your mind and be ready for a restful slumber. You can use this exercise before bed or during the day, if you find your thoughts are clouding your performance at work or you feel tired, 15 minutes of doing this exercise will add more quality to the rest of your day.

i. Loosen clothing and ensure you are in a safe environment and not driving or doing any important work.

ii. ii. Sit or lie down comfortably, preferably in a quiet place and close your eyes.

iii. Now fill your lungs with a deep breath, hold it, hold it, hold it, and then release. Repeat a few more times.

iv. Shift your attention to your feet, toes and legs: squeeze all the muscles as tight as you can, hold it, hold it, hold it and then release.

v. See how it feels to relax and let go of all the tension in your feet and legs.

vi. Now, tighten all the muscles of your thighs, hips and buttocks; hold the tension as much as you can. And then relax: feel the melting of all the tension in hips and thighs; savour the sensation of relaxation.

vii. Now, focus your attention on your neck, shoulders and back, then move down to your feet and legs. Squeeze all the muscles as tight as you can, hold it, hold it, hold it and then release the tension. See how it feels to relax and let go of all the tension in your feet and legs. Release, relax and let go.

viii. Now, fill your lungs with a deep breath – hold it, hold it, and hold and then breath out. Repeat a few more times.

ix. Now, squeeze your tummy and push your naval towards the spine. Hold as much as you can and then relax; feel the melting of the tension from your abdomen.

x. Next, raise your eyebrows, smile strongly, clench your teeth and hold it, hold it, hold it and then release the tension, relax your jaw, cheeks, eyebrows and feel blood warming up your face.

xi.   Now, imagine tensing your scalp and holding the tension for 1, 2, 3 and then releasing it. Release, relax and let go.

xii.   Notice your entire body now from head to toe. Release any remaining tension that you may be holding: your scalp, face, neck and shoulders. Release and relax your chest, tummy, your hips, thighs, feet and toes; relax.

xiii.   Enjoy the sense of ease, calm and peace.

Repeat these steps until you find ease and comfort in mind and body. Let any tension drain out of your body, beginning at the feet and slowly moving up.

Client Success Story

One of my clients, Mr Smith, could not sleep after 2am every night for nearly five months as he was launching a new product for his business and there was anxiety associated with the launch, suppliers, resources and team, in addition to worry about the success of the product and all the financial investment.

He was under the impression that this lack of sleep was normal and it would pass away. However, without realising it, this soon became the new routine for him, and his body was responding to this stress with excessive sleepiness in the afternoons. He was reaching for more sugary snacks to keep up with constant hunger and literally being fuelled by 5–6 cups of coffee in a day or sometimes even more. Mr Smith knew something needed to be changed as his doctor had recently diagnosed him with pre-diabetes, and knowing the complications of diabetes he was determined to create a positive shift in his mind and lifestyle.

We focused only on one change for the initial month: getting good quality sleep!

With the same suggestions I have shared here with you, Mr Smith transformed his sleep quality and experienced a positive effect on all other lifestyle factors: diet, more energy for exercise and activity, contentment, his weight, performance and productivity at work.

His blood check after three months showed a reduction in blood glucose, and his pre-diabetes was reversed.

"A good laugh and a long sleep are the
two best cures for anything."
—Irish proverb

SECTION 3

Mindset

"The greatest victory you can win is over your own mind."

—Swami Satchidananda

CHAPTER 9

Health Behavioural Changes

Congratulations, you are now well-equipped to create a positive lifestyle that will lead you to your desired health goals. You have envisioned how your life will positively change once you achieve your optimum health and wellness dream. You have removed negative beliefs and infused yourself with positive traits of gratitude and appreciation for your life's many blessings. You have also learned what lifestyle tools will nourish your health. Now, the real key is to use this knowledge in your daily routine and habits. Otherwise, this will be just another piece of information that you have consumed without action.

I wish long-lasting transformation for you. However, without consistent daily implementations of the tools we have discussed, it is not possible. For long-term success in your health and wellness, Daily Lifestyle Practices (DLPs) create a compounding effect and therefore incremental progress that generates a positive health gain over a period of time.

The concept of compounding is well known in the financial world. To illustrate this concept let me share an example. If you invest £10,000 at a 5% return, after a year you'll be £500 richer. Simple! But if you keep reinvesting that small profit, after ten years you will achieve a capital of £16,000; after twenty years an impressive £26,000; and after fifty, an incredible £115,000. Your money will increase exponentially.

When it comes to achieving vital health and happiness, **DLPs** are your capital because knowledge without action is merely an illusion. With daily activities, you will get small wins; as a result of those wins your confidence will soar, which will further inspire you to continue your positive lifestyle. As a result, you will get closer to achieving your desired health and wellness goals.

*"It's not that I'm so smart, it's just that
I stay with problems longer."*
—Albert Einstein

Health Behaviour Psychology

Consider this scenario: for over two decades, you have been working for long days, neglecting to connect with your family and friends, coming home to have dinner in front of the TV, before crashing in your bed.

But because of a recent health scare, you visited your general physician, who said: "Unless you change your lifestyle, eat better and exercise more, you will end up in the hospital." This threat made you feel motivated to make positive changes.

So you have started:

- Going to the gym three times a week or running outside in the winter (as opposed to being your usual complete couch potato).
- Connecting and calling your family/friends on a daily or weekly basis, while in the past many months passed by before you realised you had a social life.
- Cooking at home five days a week, instead of your daily takeaway or microwave dinners.

How long do you think these new positive changes will last? It is highly likely that you will stop that regular call or hitting the gym after your willpower is being tested by work or life demands.

What do you think the longevity of these new changes will be? One, two or three months?

If you wish to make a smooth transition integrating your new habit into your new positive lifestyle, you may need to take a different approach than making sudden changes based on pure willpower.

Here are eight principles based on the psychology of behavioural change that will help you to stay inspired to take consistent action.

Eight Behavioural Change Principles

1. Your Vision and "Why": Your vision and your reason "why" are the secret ingredients that will pull you towards consistent actions – especially when you hit an obstacle, like stress in your relationships or at work.

So really tune in to your vision and reasons daily (refer back to the visualisation exercises in the earlier chapters). Feel your dream becoming a reality: a slender body, control of your sugar levels, reversing diabetes, a younger heart age, a life filled with joy and happiness. Consistent envisioning will inspire you towards your dreams. Write your health vision as if it is already a reality. The process is powerful as when nourished by supportive, positive thoughts and actions, your subconscious brain will work towards making your health vision your reality.

Vision examples:

- I have balanced sugar levels.
- I am happy at my ideal weight of ___
- I look and feel ten years younger.
- My heart age is 30.

2. The Right Strategy: What lifestyle strategy, eating style, relaxation techniques will suit your uniqueness? Do not fall into the trap of a specific diet plan that may have worked for your friend, Tom or Susie; they are different people. Seek professional help if you need to or listen to your mind and body before creating an effective strategy to give you a long-lasting health transformation.

3. Known to Unknown: Human beings often prefer familiarity and resist the fear of the unknown.

If your new positive lifestyle behaviours are not part of your routine, then there is a vast internal resistance, and therefore any recent change you make will be temporary. Leverage existing habits and use them as a trigger to new behaviour. This way, your brain will associate familiarity with new changes, making it more likely for you to stick with the changes.

Example:

1. Use brushing your teeth as a trigger to do ten push-ups.
2. Do your gratitude journal with your morning cup of tea.
3. Use your evening commute to connect with parents or friends.
4. Use your lunch break to connect with your colleagues informally.

I invite you to brainstorm the ways you can integrate new health behaviour into your existing habits.

Exercise

Existing habits	New behaviours

4. Start with one change

Science has proven that introducing only one change at a time is more effective than trying to adopt different behavioural changes at the same time for any new changes to become our habits. Our brains cannot process too much new information at the same time. Instead of overcommitting to too many changes, give yourself a break, start with one difference, perhaps waking up 15 minutes early. Once you are successful in that, start with exercising or journaling.

Exercise:

Brainstorm all the positive health changes you wish to make and choose one change you can start right now.

1. Write a gratitude journal.
2. Start a food diary.
3. 10-minute power walk.
4.
5.

5. Start Easy

According to B J Fogg, a behavioural scientist from Stanford University, our brain perceives more challenging tasks (new lifestyle changes) as being too much effort, and therefore we are less likely to complete them. (1)

To overcome this challenge, we can trick our brains by making new changes easier. For example, when Mr Fogg wanted to start flossing his teeth, he started with flossing one tooth, triggered by brushing his teeth. In a few days, he started flossing all his teeth.

Exercise:

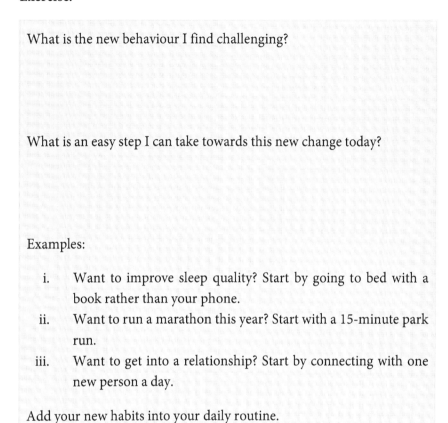

What is the new behaviour I find challenging?

What is an easy step I can take towards this new change today?

Examples:

i.   Want to improve sleep quality? Start by going to bed with a book rather than your phone.

ii. Want to run a marathon this year? Start with a 15-minute park run.

iii. Want to get into a relationship? Start by connecting with one new person a day.

Add your new habits into your daily routine.

<u>*Ease is the key for sustainability!*</u>

6. Start Now

The great philosopher and well-known author of "The Power Of Now", Eckhart Tolle believes that people have the illusion that they control their future, but this illusion only brings pain and suffering.(2) There is incredible power in the present moment. If you decide to make a change, why wait? Start today – start Now!

Give up feasting on food during Christmas telling yourself, "I will go on a diet from the new year." Instead, empower yourself by starting NOW. Please do not wait for your dream to make it a reality; start with one change, and soon the domino effect of that change will give you a positive momentum, driving you towards your ultimate health destination!

7. Habit tracker

> *"Excellence is what you repeatedly do. Excellence is not an event – it is a habit."*
> —Aristotle

Habit tracker will assist you in measuring your success by tracking your new lifestyle changes. It will act as an inspirational tool, knowing that you are making daily advancements. You can reward yourself after a period of consistent action. Just like a toddler who beams with the excitement of Brownie points or stars in their calendar, we adults as well can receive joy from this simple motivational tool.

There are different theories on the duration of making new habits; some say you have to continue new behaviour for 21 days, while UCL research suggests it takes at least 90 days to transform a habit. Irrespective of these differences, the central principle is the same: perform the new behaviour DAILY.

Exercise

As a gift to my readers, I have created a habit tracker. Download it here: https://pranitavitality.com/resources/

8. Accountability Buddy

Research in health behaviour psychology confirms the importance of accountability. According to a study by The American Society of Training and Development (ASTD), having a specific accountability partner can increase your chance of success up to 95%.(3)

When we tell someone our goal, who can keep us accountable, cheering our success and sometimes lovingly pushing us to correct and act if we fail to sustain our habits, we are more likely to make positive changes.

Right now, make a list of 5 people who can be your accountability buddies to accomplish your goals.

1.

2.

3.

4.

5.

I recommend that you join the Facebook page of this book where you can meet other likeminded readers who are aspiring to lead a positive lifestyle. You can share notes, struggles and celebrate the wins together.

"Surround yourself with people who remind you more of your future than your past."
—Dan Sullivan, a founder of Strategic Coach

CHAPTER 10

Positive Mindset

Now you have become clear on your health vision and have completed your inner work, you are READY to take consistent action on your healthy lifestyle. However, I have observed that when we are generally feeling well, it is easier to take consistent actions. Still, our negative mood and feelings often disempower us from taking actions daily.

Here, I am sharing a few tools that have helped my clients and I to shift from the negative states of being anxious, feeling low or depressed to possibility, optimism, and hope for a positive future. Their regular practise will accelerate your determination to continue on a positive path.

*Remember these tools are not a replacement for professional support. If you are experiencing consistent negative mindset and emotions, seek guidance from your health professional.

1. Cognitive Behavioural Therapy (CBT)

We often think that certain situations cause us to behave in a particular manner.

For example, you may think 'A fight with my spouse makes me angry,' (situation), 'and then I smoke/drink/overeat' (behaviour).

<u>But there is a missing link between situation and behaviour.</u>

Instead of the situation, our conscious or unconscious, positive OR negative thoughts after the situation generate reflective emotions that trigger our behaviour, healthy or harmful.

Because of the above differences in thought interpretation, one employee will argue over a colleague's disagreement. At the same time, another colleague will leave the situation for some time, take a walk and come back when he has composed himself into a productive frame of mind for a positive discussion. It's the difference in their interpretation of the situation and its related thoughts and emotions that creates these two different responses. In essence, change your thoughts to positive ones, and your behaviour and results will change automatically.

Three steps to make a change:

- The trick is to become aware of common negative thought traps.
- Pause and affirm: "I have the power to change."
- Choose alternative thoughts to overcome the negative traps.

These are examples of some of the common negative traps as described in CBT.

Negative Thinking Traps

All-or-nothing: "I have blown it. I ate one sweet; I might as well have 10."

You can find middle ground, it is not black and white.

Alternative: "It's ok, it's not the end of the world that I had one sweet. Let me go out of the room and call a friend."

Labelling: "I am lazy/fat/lonely/any other label you give to yourself."

What emotions do these negative identifying thoughts generate: empowering or disempowering?

Human beings act consistently with their own identity. So choose a different identity rather than negative labelling.

Alternative: "I am learning to make changes; I am lighter/slender/healthy/happy."

Catastrophising: "If I don't lose 10kg, I will have a heart attack, or people will reject me."

Alternative: "I am only human, and people are generally supportive. I will look for the positives in myself and other people."

Minimising/discounting positives: "My boss said 'Excellent!' But he is nice to everyone."

Acknowledge your success.

Alternative: "Well done me! I am a great asset to my organisation."

Should/Must: "I should never give way to my urges; I must go on a strict diet."

When we change "should" to "want" or "would like to,"
we feel more empowered.

Alternative: "I want to adopt a positive lifestyle that is part of my routine."

Fortune-telling /mind-reading: "I will fail in this new change."/ "He thinks that I am a bad employee."

You are either creating your future from your past experiences or imagining other people's thoughts as valid. These thoughts will cause pain and discomfort.

Alternative: "I will focus on my current activities and give my 100% to them."

"I don't know what my spouse thinks unless I speak to him."

Emotional reasoning: "I feel disgusting, so I must have gained weight."

Is it really true?

Alternative: "My feelings can change by my focus on positives; I work on feeling better."

Overgeneralisation: "I always get it wrong/am late/shout."

No, you are not: you have the power to change.

Alternative: "I was late in the past, but I have the power to manage my time better now."

Personalisation: "It's my fault that our family argued."

Self-blame does not accomplish anything positive,
so choose wisely.

Alternative: "I am only one person in the unit; together, we will move forward."

As we become aware of negative thought traps and modify them by expressing self-compassionate thoughts, we will enhance our happiness and increase our chances of success in leading a positive lifestyle.

2. Journaling

When you give your living racing thoughts, especially those of a negative nature, a channel for expression through writing, your thoughts sit beautifully in the journal rather than occupying your precious mind space.

Many creative professionals, business owners, and people interested in progressing their life forward have found journaling a useful tool to calm the mind, capture inspiration and unique ideas, and create a better future.

For this tool to be useful, I would suggest scheduling 10 minutes in the morning and 10 minutes at night to write your journal.

The following are a few questions/suggestions to guide your journaling process. However, feel free to invent and use your own unique ways to enhance a sense of ease, peace, and contentment for yourself.

Morning questions/suggestions:

1. Gratitude: write down 3 things you are grateful for today.

2. The recollection of dreams: pleasant or otherwise. Dreams serve a therapeutic purpose and sometimes give us intuitive guidance on our current life objectives or challenges we are experiencing during the day. Noting them may be a worthwhile experience for your clarity and wellness.

3. Write your essential goals for life/year/week and write three action steps you can take today that would move you towards fulfilling those goals.

4. Write your intention/s for the day ahead: Write down 1–3 emotions you wish to feel throughout the day. Remember, your intentions have immense creative power. Importantly, reaffirm those emotions throughout the day to keep yourself in a positive state.

   Some of the emotions I often pen down are:

   Bliss, Loved, Happy, Inspiring, Fulfilled, Focus, Powerful, Passionate, Purposeful, Creative, Empowering …

5. Prayer: Ask for the assistance of a higher power for a project, goals, or desires you may have.

Night:

a. Achievement of the day: note one success you experienced today, no matter how small or big; you will sleep with a sense of accomplishment.

b. Key learnings of the day: so that you can better yourself daily, incrementally.

c. Set an intention: "I enjoy sound and rejuvenating sleep for a successful, energised, and productive tomorrow."

d. Write any thoughts that create anxiety or worry on one side of the paper, and on the other side, write what action steps you can take and when you would do them. This is very powerful as you are putting your brain at ease, knowing that important matters will be addressed in time; your subconscious mind can feel at ease and relax.

3. Boxed breathing

A breathing exercise to release overthinking, anxiety, or worry.

People find it challenging to stick to positive behaviour because they are often ruminating or anxious about some other areas of their lives. A specific breathing exercise called Boxed Breathing will help you to calm your nerves and sustain positive behaviour, including deep, restful sleep.

- Make yourself comfortable by sitting or lying down.
- Close your eyes and focus on your breathing, releasing all other thoughts.
- Breathe in for the count of 4, hold for seven and breath out for a count of 8.
- Do this a few times, focusing on breathing, noticing the warmth of your breath as it passes through your lungs, and relaxes your body.
- Breathe in for the count of 4, hold for seven, and breathe out for a count of 8.
- Repeat until you feel calm.

4. Appreciate and celebrate your wins

Make these words your new vocabulary: "Well done! Amazing! Excellent! Bravo!"

When you are learning to adopt a new behaviour, for example, choosing a snack of fruit or salad rather than eating a cookie or drinking herbal tea rather than ordering coffee, it is a habit change. Every small win should be acknowledged.

When a baby is learning to walk and fall, we do not criticise the baby and say, "You will never be able to walk," but instead, we use gentle words of encouragement. Use the same approach when you are making positive changes. Instead of criticising our small mistakes and setbacks, say phrases such as:

> "I am learning to adopt positive habits; every day it gets easier for me to make changes" or

> "I am releasing the old habits and accepting the new one/s with ease."

You can also look at the other areas of your life where you already feel empowered: maybe you have a successful career or are an excellent parent. Now, the affirmation could be:

> "I am already a success in _____. Therefore, I could be successful in my health journey as well. I have the confidence to create a positive shift in all areas of my life."

The Temporal Theory of Motivation confirms two factors that determine the sustained motivation for positive changes: firstly, the value of the result you want to achieve (your WHY), and secondly, your self-belief in your ability to achieve the goal.(4) That means if weight loss is absolutely necessary for you like you have a gun to your head and you have to lose that excess 10 kg, then provided that you have a strong belief system, you will maintain the positive changes and soon will achieve the result. Celebrating small wins and affirming your abilities to achieve success will help you enhance your self-belief, self-efficacy, and confidence to change your new identity positively.

Rome was not built in a day, so be patient with yourself. Ask yourself, "What is the one small action I can do towards my health goal?"

Brainstorm a few ideas and act on them. A few small changes – a 10-minute walk, talk to your friend to get support, choose a carrot stick snack instead of a cookie – will all add up to build your confidence muscle, and soon this new behaviour will become easier to sustain. Even if today all you managed to do was to become aware of your mental chatter and noted this in your diary, you are already different from the majority of the population living life on autopilot, unconscious of their thoughts and behaviour. *Well done!*

Mirror technique to enhance self-belief: Say something positive about yourself every time you pass the mirror, or you could verbalise your affirmations, your positive qualities while looking into your eyes. This simple technique will catapult your level of confidence in achieving your health goals.

5. Celebrate

Keep up your health commitment by tuning in to your vision, listening to inspirational podcasts, and being around positive people. Reward yourself on small achievements. When you celebrate your journey, you will be able to ENJOY the process towards a happy and healthy heart.

I have written a list of celebration ideas you may consider and (add your own) to reward yourself for accomplishing your goals.

Celebration /rewards for consistent lifestyle actions.

- Spa day.
- Massage.
- Watch a movie with your sweetheart or a good friend.
- Dinner at your favourite restaurant.

These are just some of the ways to enhance your emotional wellness and positive mindset. However, there are various other tools available, and each works differently for different personalities. I received tremendous benefits from therapies such as Reiki and Emotional Freedom Techniques, and I would encourage you to read about them and work with a specific practitioner to benefit from them. Your objective is to continue to feel a sense of ease and happiness.

As you progress through various stages of life, your definition of success and happiness will evolve. The key is to be mindful of the changes and continuously strive to improve your emotions. Various tools described throughout this book will help you to achieve a sense of wellness. You can easily fulfil any goals from that happy place, including your health goals of a slender body, optimum health, and VITALITY.

This is my wish for you.

SECTION 4

What Really Matters

"The purpose of our lives is to be happy"
—His Holiness Dalai Lama

CHAPTER 11

Happiness: Connection

What is Happiness?

I believe living a genuinely happy life means living a connected life. This means savouring a deeper bond with others, by living in awareness and alignment with our true values and purpose, and relating with another being with empathy, deep compassion, understanding, nonjudgment, and acceptance in the spirit of unconditional love.

To contribute to others' wellness, we have to ensure we are filled with love, respect, and compassion for ourselves. A growing body of science shows the importance of mindfulness, breathwork, and meditation in strengthening this connection at the mind-body-spirit level.

When we engage in these practices, we experience a release of negative thoughts and emotions that keep us stuck in the past hurts and traumas, and release anxiety about the future (fear of debt, being alone, dying). Throughout this book, we have learned practices such as visualisation, forgiveness exercises, yoga, and conscious breathing. These practices help us bring our attention to the present moment, where our real power lies, where we can experience pure bliss and internal joy; we can tap into our creativity and an exponential power intuition.

Benefits of meditation on health and wellness

- **Improves heart function:** Meditation assists with reducing blood pressure in people with hypertension and it also lowers high cholesterol levels. A systematic review published in 2007 assessed several methods of stress reduction in patients with hypertension and found satisfactory benefits (i.e., 5/3 mm Hg systolic/diastolic blood pressure reduction) with the practice of meditation.(1)

Even esteemed scientific organisations are recognising the importance of meditation. A scientific statement from the American Heart Association reviews numerous studies on meditation and acknowledges this low-risk intervention in reducing cardiovascular disease risk factors.(2)

- **Decreased anxiety, depression, and insomnia**: A pivotal study led by scientists at the University of California, San Francisco, found that participants who underwent a short, intensive meditation program were less depressed, anxious, and stressed, while also experiencing positive emotional traits (beneficial for social connection) such as greater compassion and awareness of others' feelings. (3)

- **Reduction in stress:** The regular practice of meditation reduces the production of "stress hormones," including cortisol and adrenaline. The body releases stress hormones due to the flight-or-fight response, our survival mechanism. It is meant to prompt us to run away from the danger of being eaten by a lion in the wild. However, many modern-day experiences (being stuck in the traffic, unhappy work environment, frustrations with spouse or kids) can produce the same bodily response. It releases stress hormones, reduces the blood supply to our digestive organs, and diverts blood to our legs instead in preparation to run away from danger. It also causes our body to speed up our heart rate, increase our blood sugar, suppress our immune system, and reduce insulin production.

Over time, this causes cumulative negative changes to the functioning of essential organs' responses. Many compelling studies are showing the power of meditation to relieve stress and promote inner calm. For example, a 2011 study (RCT) published in the *Evidence-Based Complementary and Alternative Medicine Journal* found that full-time workers who spent a few hours each week practising mindfulness meditation reported a significant decrease in job stress, anxiety, and depressed mood. (4)

- **Enhances cognitive skills:** Increasing cognitive skills such as focus, attention span, learning, and memory, are beneficial for our business, career, and financial wellness. A recent study led by researchers from Harvard University found that after only eight weeks of meditation, participants experienced healthy growth in the grey matter of the brain in the areas associated with memory, learning, empathy, self-awareness, and stress regulation. This study also demonstrates the brain's remarkable plasticity and ability to change habitual stress responses. (5)

- **Enhances creativity and intuition:** With meditation, we focus on creating the space by disengaging from the constant stream of thoughts and internal dialogue. A pioneer in integrative medicine, Dr Deepak Chopra, describes this state as "Pure Potentiality" where we expand our awareness and tap into intuition, insights, and fresh ideas. Many high achievers in various fields – scientists, athletes, top professionals, entrepreneurs, term this state as being in 'FLOW'. Flowing without resistance, you accomplish more with ease rather than struggle.

Meditation Practices

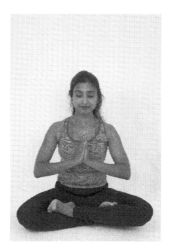

While there are many practices I have learned over the period, which benefited me and those with whom I shared them, there are a few that I will describe here for their simplicity. I encourage you to try them. Use the one that resonates most with you or is most to your liking.

A vital thing to consider before entering into any style of meditation is to relax your physical body. One way to do this is a practice of progressive muscle relaxation, discussed in an earlier chapter on sleep, where you tense and relax your body to induce a state of deep relaxation. Alternatively, you can also choose to meditate immediately after waking up when your body and mind are relaxed.

Breath Awareness Meditation

Sit in a quiet place, wearing comfortable clothes, with soothing lights, away from the outside world's distraction and noise, either in a chair or on the mat on the floor, wherever you feel comfortable.

Now with eyes closed, relax your body and bring your attention to your breath. As you observe the breath, you will notice it will slow down automatically. Keep observing your breath; if your mind wanders for a few moments, notice it and slowly bring it back to your breathing.

Gradually, you will notice that thoughts are fading away like clouds passing in a clear blue sky. You will clear clouds of thoughts to clear your consciousness and move into a positive state of being. You will experience a state of restful awareness.

Transcendental Meditation:

If focusing on just breathing is difficult for you, you can also focus on repeating a word. In Indian spiritual practices, the term 'OM' is repeated as it produces positive vibration throughout your body. You can choose any word depending on your belief system. You can even choose to repeat the positive emotions you wish to cultivate, such as: love, gratitude, and bliss. Or simply focus on one song or[6] binaural beats.

Guided Meditation and Visualisation:

If you are new to meditation, guided practice will make your journey more comfortable, as you are gently guided by a practitioner to achieve a sense of silence and peace. This method is also useful if you experience specific issues such as anger towards a situation or a person, feeling sad or anxious, or overcoming a particular health challenge.

You can use visualisations we discussed earlier in the book; ideal health visualisations, forgiveness, and positive states like love and gratitude. You can also use visualisation to create the positive experience you desire in the present moment, such as a visualisation for being disease-free, healthy, happy and being at an ideal weight.

---

[6] Binaural beat therapy is an emerging form of sound wave therapy.

Here, I share one such guided practice for enhancing happiness in your heart.

Meditation for a Happy Heart

When our minds and hearts are filled with positive emotions for various aspects of our lives, we tend to see the light of hope, even in the darkest mental distress. Reflecting on emotions such as appreciation, gratitude, and the joy and love surrounding you, melts away fear, anxiety, or sadness.

This meditation has lifted me multiple times to overcome stresses and sadness and become hopeful and optimistic.

It is best to do this meditation first thing in the morning to set your day off on a positive note. But you can do this meditation at any time of day when you need to improve your emotional state.

- Place yourself in any comfortable position sitting or lying down.

- Now, close your eyes and connect with your breath.

- Imagine breathing in relaxation and breathing out tension.

- You may notice your mind is calmer, and your heartbeat is slower.

- Just enjoy the warm feeling of peace throughout your body as a wave of breathing warms your entire body.

- Now, observe your heart and breathe deep into your heart, and notice blood flowing through your heart and nourishing your whole body. Notice your heart's strength – the love and compassion of your heart that it possesses for all other beings; feel and appreciate this gift of life.

- Feel grateful for the personal qualities that you admire and appreciate about yourself.

- As you appreciate your heart, picture any person in your life who you love and respect. It can be any person – this may be your child, your parent, a dear friend, or even a stranger who said words of encouragement to you. What about that person you love the most? Feel those emotions right now – their presence, support, unconditional love, wisdom, guidance, or anything that comes in your mind.

- Now bring to mind any situation/s that you feel immensely grateful for. This may be a blissful sunrise, natural beauty, life lessons or coincidences that have positively influenced your life somehow.

- Now, set the intention to improve positive feelings of mental strength, appreciation, love, creativity, joy, and allow these to flow into your consciousness. Feel this shift is happening right now, feel the sense of accomplishment, celebrate with a smile.

- Notice the sensation in your heart.

- Know that you can come back to this highest emotional state at any time you wish.

- Spend a few moments in these feelings before gently opening your eyes.

"Water is fluid, soft and yielding. But water will wear away rock, which is rigid and cannot yield. As a rule, whatever is fluid, soft and yielding will overcome whatever is rigid and hard. This is another paradox: what is soft is strong."
—Lau Tzu

CHAPTER 12

Happiness: Contribution

With the practices described throughout the book, you will create a stillness within you, a space without anger, resentment, and hate, filled with a purity of forgiveness, non-judgment, love, and compassion for everyone around you. From this space, it is possible for you to form new relationships and strengthen your existing friendship bonds, based on mutual respect, growth, and love. Once you feel strong in your mind and body, and are aligned with your unique values, you will contribute to humanity with your unique purpose. **A sense of contribution to your family, community, clients, and broader society will bring your happiness to the next level.**

Exercise to improve connection with others.

1. Make a list of your connections: friends, colleagues, acquaintances.

2. Make a plan to reach out to them from the space of love and compassion.

3. How are you going to express your love?
    - A letter or a greeting card.
    - A gift: small or big.
    - Flowers.
    - A call.
    - Meet for a coffee or a meal.
    - Bond over activities or travel.

Creating New Connections:

If you are new to the area, explore how you can form new friendships.

These are a few suggestions:

- Join a health club.
- Join a Meetup group you are interested in.
- Go to a business or professional networking event.
- If you are a parent, reach out to another parent for a coffee and/or a play date.
- Volunteer at a local charity shop where you can meet new people while helping the community.
- Help people in your neighbourhood.
- Host a party for your neighbours.

Try to create value in each of your encounters with new people.

- What would you add to this list?............

> *"Possibilities are endless; you only need an intent to connect with a pure heart."*
> —Pranita Salunke

Purpose

> *"Purpose is the life-giving blood for our existence."*
> —Pranita Salunke

When we are engaged in meaningful activities that give us a sense of identity and fulfilment, we feel secure, content and happy. While working in rehabilitation units (as an Occupational Therapist), I observed that becoming independent, even in a simple task of self-care like washing and dressing, gave an immense sense of purpose and achievement for people recovering from major illnesses or surgery.

In his book, "The Blue Zones: Lessons for Living Longer From the People Who've Lived the Longest", author Dan Buettner observes that the presence of a strong sense of 'purpose' has helped specific communities in Japan to live a longer and healthier life.(6)

The term 'IKIGAI' (or purpose) in the Japanese tradition means: a reason to be, the reason for existence, expressing your unique talents and gifts and creativity for your fulfilment and society.

Your purpose is seen in action in various ways. When a mum is singing a lullaby to her baby; when grandma is cooking a Sunday meal for her family; when an entrepreneur is presenting his vision to his team; when a volunteer is working to support his cause, or when a dedicated teacher is shaping the future of our next generation with her teachings and unique manners!

Strong evidence suggests the importance of having a sense of meaning and purpose of physical and mental health. The result from a survey conducted at Oregon State University showed that irrespective of previous health conditions, when people retired at age 66 instead of 65, their death rates dropped by a full 11%. The meaningful work and economic and social benefits of working for one more life year could contribute to this positive result.(7) For people who are career-driven work is part of their identity, and if they retire early they have a greater chance of suffering from ill-health and premature death. A study published in the National Bureau of Economic Research found a two per cent increase in the male death rate immediately after age 62 when they retired early. Loss of identity, reduced social interactions, and financial pressures are potential reasons for this decline.(8)

Personally, I feel more alert, healthier, and happier when I am engaged in meaningful work; either writing, speaking, working with my clients, and fulfilling my duties as a mum or as a daughter. All these roles give me a sense of identity and meaning, bring out the best in me, help me work on my weaknesses, evolve me into a better human, a better person – and that feeling, my friends, is priceless!

Indian philosophy also promotes the value of 'KARM-Yoga – a Yoga of action' as one of the essential paths towards fulfilment and spiritual liberation.

If you are leading a purposeful life already, that is great. Keep up the excellent work! However, if you are at a life stage where you wish to get a fresher perspective of your life's purpose, an exercise to explore your purpose and live it daily could enhance your health and happiness levels.

An exercise I often recommend to my clients to find is the 'Ikigai Model' that helps them explore their real purpose. The model is best described by four overlapping circles representing your passion, mission, calling, and career. The place where the four processes meet is where you find your 'ikigai'. Here I share this exercise with some of the questions that will assist you in finding your IKIAGI. You can choose to answer the following questions freehand or in bullet points; the choice is yours. Get creative, put on some music, and enjoy this self-exploratory journey as I share this exercise with you.

Exercise

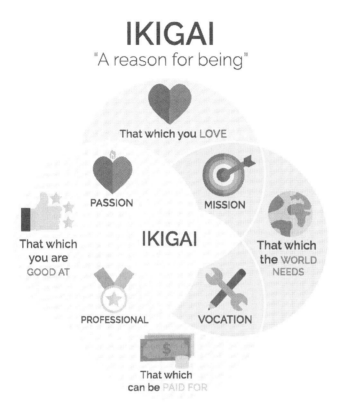

IKIGAI

"A reason for being"

That which you LOVE

PASSION

MISSION

That which you are GOOD AT

IKIGAI

That which the WORLD NEEDS

PROFESSIONAL

VOCATION

That which can be PAID FOR

What I love:

- What are my top 3 values in life?
- What does a successful, happy life look like for me?
- What brings me the most joy and sense of peace in my life?

What I am good at:

- What are my top 10 achievements in life?
- What do others most admire in me?
- What are my strengths?

What the world needs:

- What unique gifts would I like to share with the world?
- What do I want to contribute to this world?
- What legacy do I want to leave behind?

What you are/could be paid for?

- What unique gifts would I like to share with the world?
- How do I want to grow?

Additional questions to assist you in this exercise:

- Who am I?
- My understanding of the meaning of my existence.
- My life's goals, dreams, and desires?
- Three words that capture the essence of who you are or wish to be.

Once you answer, all the questions, observe any overlapping theme that comes into your awareness. What does the intersection area suggest? Maybe it's innovation, technology, teaching, business, creation, art, baking, volunteering, becoming a writer, or something else?

I welcome you to find your own IKIGAI and enjoy your unique meaningful existence on Mother Earth while leaving your true legacy.

CHAPTER 13

Conclusion

A positive lifestyle empowers us to achieve a healthy heart that beats stronger for longer. If you apply the principles outlined in this book, you will enhance your lifespan and will be able to enjoy an immensely joyful and happy life. You will be able to savour all your relationships, but you will most importantly discover and strengthen your relationship with yourself. Once your inner being is happy, you will enhance your focus, cultivate creativity, and deliver immense passion for your craft and purpose. Abundance, wealth and fulfilment is a natural result of this process.

There is a natural sequence for the application of the Vitality principles in your daily life that may help you to remember them. When a human being comes into existence, our spirit form aspires to assume a physical form; therefore, starting from a connection with yourself is of utmost importance. At an embryo stage, the foetus receives information through the surrounding cells and environment. Your mind starts developing in the womb and continues to flourish after birth with the experiences you receive as a young child. To strengthen your mindset, you need to discover your true desires and empower yourself. You can do this by identifying and replacing negative beliefs with more powerful ones through the repetition of positive affirmations. As you cultivate a powerful mindset, it will help you create a healthy and positive lifestyle – an easy walk on luscious grass. Your attitude determines your thoughts and lifestyle choices, which ultimately determine your physical and mental health.

Making these positive mind-body-connection shifts will not only help you but will also create better health for your future generations to come! Becoming aware of your health markers, adopting a positive lifestyle of using food as a source of nourishment, becoming conscious of the source and digestion of food rather than worrying about counting calories, enjoying eating mindfully, moving joyously, enjoying deep restorative sleep, and importantly, knowledge of lifestyle habit formation, will be incredibly transformative for your health and well-being.

Once you feel strong in your own body and mind, connecting and contributing to others with your unique traits, core values, and purpose will be your innate desire. Incorporating these Vitality principles, you will ultimately achieve your ideal body weight, have optimum heart health, and an inner joy that you desire and deserve.

I hope with this book, I have inspired you to believe that:

Prevention is always better than cure.

Mind, Body and Connection are three principles to achieve optimum health and vitality!

Self-Love initiates our healing journey.

A Purpose-led life is worth striving for.

Health and Happiness is the foundation for a successful life.

You are a powerful being and can achieve anything your heart desires, including optimum health, vitality, and happiness. I wish you immense joy along your beautiful journey!

Live well. Live with Vitality!

Pranita

"Knowledge is of no value unless you put it into practice."
—Anton Chekhov

CHAPTER 14

21-Day Challenge

The 21-Day Vitality Healthy and Happy Heart Challenge draws together the action steps from this book. I have created this guide to help you start your journey of lifestyle transformation by forming positive health habits. You can use the Habit Tracker to track your progress throughout your 21-day plan.
(Download it here: https://pranitavitality.com/resources/)

Day 1: Awareness is the Key to Your Transformation

Write an honest reflection on your health and wellness. Complete the Vitality Self Questionnaire which is at the beginning of the book . You may not know all the answers, for example, your blood tests. Write as much detail as possible with the date next to each entry.

After you take action on all the aspects, we have covered in this book, you can re-take the self-assessment and enjoy the feeling of success as you see the improvement in your score.

Day 2: Investigate

If you are aware of any risk factors for yourself as we discussed in Chapter 1 – diabetes, being overweight, any existing disease or severe psychological stress – perhaps you may wish to approach your health professional to assess what your current biomarkers are:

- Levels of Triglycerides
- Blood glucose
- HbA1C
- Heart Age
- Or any other tests your health professional may recommend enhancing your health awareness.

Remember, the purpose of this exercise is not to get scared with the numbers, but to use it as motivation to lead a healthy lifestyle.

Day 3: Set a Bold Vision

Get yourself a beautiful journal. On the first page of the journal, write, 'My Successful Journey to a Vital, Healthy and Happy Heart.'

On the next page, write where you are at currently in your aspirations. The work you did on Day 1 and Day 2 will help you to write the answer.

Set a grand vision for your health success that is unique to you and that inspires you to act consistently towards its fulfilment. Declare that you are now committed to: making transformation happen; to dive into your true potential; to succeed; and to create a positive shift in your world.

Write down your WHY? Why do you want to achieve success?

How will your love life change as a result of this transformation?

How will your business and career catapult when you are healthy, look, and feel good?

Write all the details about where you will be, who you would be surrounded by, what new hobbies you will take, what new destinations you would travel to? Go wild!

Write in your journal daily from now on, reflecting on your actions, insights, and ideas you may have along the journey.

Day 4: Create a Vision Board

Create a vision board by collecting images and inspirational words that convey the emotions of your visions that you set on the day.

You can get free printable inspirational quotes on the Internet – choose one that speaks to your heart. See Chapter 2.

Day 5: Visualise Your Success

Display your vision board where you can see it regularly. Some suggestions are your bedroom wall, fridge, or phone display, or you may wish to create a vision book.

Visualise daily in the morning and as you get ready to sleep.

Look at those images with inspirational music in the background. I found binaural beats or a song that brings happiness in my heart works best for this purpose.

Close your eyes and visualise yourself, achieving your health and wellness goals, and savour those emotions.

You can also download a guided health visualisation I have created for you to listen to daily. (https://pranitavitality.com/video/)

Read and practise visualisations we discussed in Chapter 2.

Day 6: Mission

Today, take time to identify your life's mission: one for life and one career or business.

What do you really want to experience in life: travel, marriage, speaking to a huge audience, dancing, learning, or growth?

Write it down, as this will fuel your inspiration to take your health to the next level.

Day 7: Purpose

Your purpose will help you to leave your unique legacy in the world.

My business purpose is: *To inspire, educate, and empower people for healthy lifestyle transformation.*

This purpose gives me focus and clarity.

Reflect on your daily job: does it awaken your true passion and give fulfilment?

Undertake the Ikigai exercise we discussed in Chapter 12 to help you identify your purpose.

Make a plan to live your Ikigai from today!

Day 8: Values are the Compass for Your life.

The self-reflective exercise from the Ikigai principle will also help you identify your core values and beliefs about life and business.

My own business values are:
Compassionate care
Professionalism
My clients' success

Write down your values for business and life.

Day 9: Create a Plan

Now you know your life's vision, purpose, and values.

Create your health and wellness goal that will fuel your BIG LIFE VISION.

Chunk down your health goal into easily manageable steps.

Ask yourself:

- What needs to be changed?
- Who will support me in achieving my health goals?
- What resources will I need: books, online, people?
- What actions do I need to take?

Put those actions in the calendar. Start taking action today!

Day 10: Observe Your Thoughts and Emotions

Emotional wellness is the key to take sustained action steps that will lead you to your destination.

If you are consistently feeling any negative emotions, become aware of your feelings, and name those emotions:
anger/frustration/sadness/stress.

Try to find the source of the pain. You can use some of the tools we discussed in the book to manage your emotions, such as Cognitive Behavioural Therapy. (Chapter 10)

However, sometimes you may need to reach for support. I recommend reading "Heal your Life" by Louise Hay and also take professional support to help you achieve emotional wellness if you need some close hand-holding in your journey to optimum health.

Day 11: Start a Meditation Practice of Your Choice

Meditation is a powerful tool to help you manage your emotions and achieve a level of happiness.

Start to experiment with various tools and meditations we have discussed in this book and from other resources until you identify the one that suits you the most.

Day 12: Nourishing Food

Start a food diary to help you become aware of how your daily meals and drinks and thoughts create your current health, weight, digestive issues, and energy levels.

After reading about Nourishment (in Chapter 6) and evaluating your food diary, you can start removing the food items that do not serve your health goals.

Find your free printable food and lifestyle diary here: link https://pranitavitality.com/resources/

Day 13: Prepare for Rejuvenation

Prepare for rejuvenation with real, wholesome foods that we explored in the nutrition sections and perhaps invest in kitchen appliances to help make your cooking experience more enjoyable. These include good quality cast iron utensils, juicers, blenders, etc.

Make a weekly healthy meal plan with your family and shop beforehand so that you are prepared to enjoy optimum health and vitality.

Use the recipes mentioned here for inspiration, or there are a few other recipes in the healthy weight guide I have created – you can download the guide here: https://pranitavitality.com/resources/

Day 14: Joyful Movement

Bring awareness into your current activity levels; a 3-day diary will assist you with this.

Now you are committed to a positive transformation, make a list of all the ways you can start becoming more active in your current routine. For example, a walk in between your meetings or during your lunch break, standing during sessions instead of sitting down. Write down your plan and start taking action today.

Day 15: Fitness

Today, make a list of fitness activities you enjoy. Maybe you love the buzz of group exercise, such as aerobics, dance, strength training? Research the club or gym that offers what you like and join it today.

If you prefer a more social way of keeping active, look up sports clubs of your choice: football, cricket, golf, or rugby.

See Chapter 7: Joyful Movement.

Day 16: Sleep

Bring awareness into your current activity levels by noting your sleep quality and quantity. Your 3-day and sleep diary will assist you with this. (See Chapter 8)

Remove any barriers preventing you from a good quality sleep; invest in a quality mattress or a white noise playlist.

Good quality sleep will ensure you are recovering from the mental and physical stresses you are experiencing daily.

Day 17: Contact your Health Professional

If you have identified any sleep issues such as sleep apnoea (or any other concern as you progress), arrange an appointment with your health care professional for getting help today.

Day 18: Connections and friendship

Cultivate meaningful friendships by reaching out to your friends, neighbours, and even online groups.

Social connection is the secret sauce for our happiness. So, make a list of all the people you can connect with and share your joy, pain, and listen to theirs.

Speak to them with the love, compassion, and empathy you like to receive. Message or call one of them today and enjoy the magic of connection.

Join online groups where you can meet people with the same goals and vision. They may have an in-person event to attend, or connect with an individual member you feel comfortable with to form an accountability buddy.

If you wish to be part of my community, I would love to welcome you. You can find more at:
https://www.facebook.com/Pranitavitality
https://www.linkedin.com/in/pranita-salunke-9a92873a/

Day 19: Contribution

A life of meaning is a life worth living.

When you are enjoying optimum health and vitality, you want to share that joy in the world with your purposeful endeavours; you are inspired to contribute to your family, friends, and community.

Write five things you can do to contribute to your loved ones and start taking action, even if this means reaching out to one friend in need and listening with a compassionate heart.

Day 20: Reflect

Hurray, you are almost at the end of your challenge. I hope you are now inspired and have progressed over the past 20 days.

To conclude, I would like you to journal your achievements and learnings for the past 20 days. Write about your joy, insights, aha moments, wins you may have!

Day 21: Celebrate!

Celebrate your successes, however small or large they may be. Wins, when celebrated, will reinforce your neurology to continue on your healthy lifestyle journey.

Well done for sticking to the path, I am very proud of you.

Write three things, people, and experiences you are grateful for over these last 21 days. Express your gratitude in person with these people.

Continue the positive journey beyond this point with a firm intention of leading a vital, healthy, and happy life!

You have my loving wishes with you!

Pranita

"Health and happiness are the foundation for a successful life."

—Pranita Salunke

#vitalityhealthyandhappyheart

References

Introduction

1. <u>Ed Diener</u> et al 2017. 'If, Why, and When Subjective Well-Being Influences Health, and Future Needed Research'.
   https://pubmed.ncbi.nlm.nih.gov/28707767/

2. Susan Connolly et al 2011. 'MyAction: an innovative approach to the prevention of cardiovascular disease in the community'
   https://bjcardio.co.uk/2011/08/myactionaninnovativeapproachtothep
   reventionofcardiovasculardisease/

Chapter 1: The Big Picture

1. National Health Services, September 2018.
   https://www.nhs.uk/conditions/cardiovascular-disease/

2. World Health Organisation, 2017. Cardiovascular diseases (CVDs). Retrieved from:
   https://www.who.int/cardiovascular_diseases/about_cvd/en/

3. National Health Services, September 2018.
   https://www.nhs.uk/conditions/cardiovascular-disease/

4. Sources: World Heart Federation, September 2011. Harvard School of Public Health – The Global Economic Burden of Non-communicable Diseases.
   http://www3.weforum.org/docs/WEF_Harvard_HE_GlobalEconomi
   cBurdenNonCommunicableDiseases_2011.pdf

5. World Health Organization, 2020. Noncommunicable diseases: Childhood overweight and obesity
   https://www.who.int/dietphysicalactivity/childhood/en/

6. UNICEF. (2018a). Malnutrition rates remain alarming: stunting is declining too slowly while wasting still impacts the lives of far too many young children. Retrieved from http://data.unicef.org/topic/nutrition/malnutrition/#.

7. Centers for Disease Control and Prevention, 2020. https://www.cdc.gov/coronavirus/2019-ncov/need-extra-precautions/people-with-medical-conditions.html

8. Spanakis and Golden, 2013. Race/Ethnic Difference in Diabetes and Diabetic Complications. https://www.ncbi.nlm.nih.gov/pmc/articles/PMC3830901/-diabetes-an-approach-to- implementation/ https://drhyman.com/blog/2016/04/05/is-predisposition-pre-destiny

9. Alegría-Torres and colleague, 2011. Epigenetics and Lifestyle. https://www.ncbi.nlm.nih.gov/pmc/articles/PMC3752894/

10. Dr Mark Hayman. Retrieved, 2020. https://drhyman.com/blog/2016/03/03/are-my-genes-making-me-fat-and-sick/

11. Scott, 2016. Genetic Factors Are Not the Major Causes of Chronic Diseases https://www.ncbi.nlm.nih.gov/pmc/articles/PMC4841510/

12. World Health Organisation, 2005. 'Preventing CHRONIC DISEASES a vital investment'. https://www.who.int/chp/chronic_disease_report/full_report.pdf?ua=1

13. Joint British Society, board 3, 2014. 'JBS cardiovascular disease prevention guideline'. https://www.guidelines.co.uk/cardiovascular/jbs-cardiovascular-disease-prevention- guideline/251614.article

14. National Health Services, 2016. 'What's your heart age?' https://www.nhs.uk/conditions/nhs-health-check/check-your-heart-age-tool/

15. Schneiderman et al.2005. 'STRESS AND HEALTH: Psychological, Behavioural, and Biological Determinants'.
https://www.ncbi.nlm.nih.gov/pmc/articles/PMC2568977/

Section 1

1. Royal Society for Public Health, 2016. 'Quitting smoking is the most difficult New Year's resolution to keep'. Retrieved from:
https://www.rsph.org.uk/about-us/news/quitting-smoking-most-difficult-new-year-s-resolution-to-keep-3-in-5-smoke-again-by-31-january.html

2. Dr Wayne W. Dyer, 'Inspiration and Purpose'. Retrieved
https://www.drwaynedyer.com/press/inspiration-purpose/

3. Dr Deepak Chopra, 'The Spontaneous Fulfilment of Desire: Harnessing the Infinite Power of Coincidence.' Harmony Books; 1st edition (1 Feb. 2004).

4. Louise L. Hay: 'You Can Heal Your Life' Hay House. 1 Jan.1984

Section 2

Nourishment

1. Wiss et al. 2018. Sugar Addiction: From Evolution to Revolution. Retrieved from:
https://www.ncbi.nlm.nih.gov/pmc/articles/PMC6234835/

2. DiNicolantonio and OKeefe, 2017. Added sugars drive coronary heart disease via insulin resistance and hyperinsulinaemia: a new paradigm.
https://www.ncbi.nlm.nih.gov/pmc/articles/PMC5708308/

3. Mozaffarian, 2017. Foods, obesity, and diabetes – are all calories created equal? https://pubmed.ncbi.nlm.nih.gov/28049747/

4. Vani Hari: 'Feeding You Lies: How to Unravel the Food Industry's Playbook and Reclaim Your Health'. Hay House Inc; 1st edition (19 Feb. 2019)
https://www.amazon.co.uk/Feeding-You-Lies-Industrys-Playbook/dp/1401954545

5. Soffritti et al. 2005; 'Aspartame induces lymphomas and leukaemias in rats.' European Journal of Oncology. Retrieved from:
http://citeseerx.ist.psu.edu/viewdoc/download?doi=10.1.1.482.6743&rep=rep1&type=pdf

6. U.S. Food and Drug Administration, 2018. 'Additional Information about High-Intensity Sweeteners Permitted for Use in Food in the United States'. Retrieved from:
https://www.fda.gov/food/food-additives-petitions/additional-information-about-high-intensitysweeteners-permitted-use-food-united-states)

7. Harvard Health Publishing, 2019. 'The truth about fats: the good, the bad, and the in-between'. https://www.health.harvard.edu/staying-healthy/the-truth-about-fats-bad-and-good

8. Harvard Health Publishing, 2019. 'The truth about fats: the good, the bad, and the in-between'. https://www.health.harvard.edu/staying-healthy/the-truth-about-fats-bad-and-good

9. European Society of Cardiology, 2016. 2016 European Guidelines on Cardiovascular Disease Prevention in Clinical Practice: The Sixth Joint Task Force of the European Society of Cardiology and Other Societies on Cardiovascular Disease Prevention in Clinical Practice.
https://academic.oup.com/eurheartj/article/37/29/2315/1748952

10. JBS 2: Joint British Societies' guidelines on prevention of cardiovascular disease in clinical practice. Retrieved from:
https://heart.bmj.com/content/91/suppl_5/v1

11. Burns 2003, BURNS, DM, Epidemiology of smoking-induced cardiovascular disease. Progress in Cardiovascular Diseases. Retrieved from: https://pubmed.ncbi.nlm.nih.gov/12920698/

12. Albakri* , 2018 'Alcoholic cardiomyopathy: A review of literature on clinical status and meta-analysis of diagnostic and clinical management methods'.
https://pubs.niaaa.nih.gov/publications/arh293/199-202.pdf).

13. Hart et al. 2010. 'The combined effect of smoking tobacco and drinking alcohol on cause-specific mortality: a 30-year cohort study'. https://bmcpublichealth.biomedcentral.com/articles/10.1186/1471-2458-10-789

14. National Health Services, 2019 'Food intolerance'. Retrieved from: https://www.nhs.uk/conditions/food-intolerance/

15. Trichopoulou et al. 2003. 'Adherence to a Mediterranean diet and survival in a Greek population'. Retrieved from:
https://www.ncbi.nlm.nih.gov/pubmed/12826634?dopt=Abstract

16. Féart et al 2011. 'Adherence to a Mediterranean diet and onset of disability in older persons.' Retrieved from:
https://link.springer.com/article/10.1007/s10654-011-9611-4

17. Kris-Etherton et al. 2001. 'Lyon Diet Heart Study. Benefits of a Mediterranean-Style, National Cholesterol Education Program/American Heart Association Step I Dietary Pattern on Cardiovascular Disease. Retrieved from:
https://www.ahajournals.org/doi/full/10.1161/01.cir.103.13.1823

18. Minich, 2019. A Review of the Science of Colorful Plant-Based Food and Practical Strategies for "Eating the Rainbow".
https://www.researchgate.net/publication/333577389_A_Review_of_the_Science_of_Colorful_Plant-Based_Food_and_Practical_Strategies_for_Eating_the_Rainbow

19. Harvard Health Publishing, 2019. Phytonutrients: Paint your plate with the colors of the rainbow. Retrieved from: https://www.health.harvard.edu/blog/phytonutrients-paint-your-plate-with-the-colors-of-the-rainbow-2019042516501

20. Honeycutt, 2017. 'Eating The Rainbow: Why Eating a Variety of Fruits and Vegetables Is Important for Optimal Health'. Retrieved from: https://foodrevolution.org/blog/eating-the-rainbow-health-benefits/

21. Jennings et al. 2009. 'Preventive Cardiology: A practical manual (Oxford Care Manuals), Oxford University Press.

22. Harvard Health Publication, 2020. 'Glycaemic index for 60+ foods'. Retrieved from: https://www.health.harvard.edu/diseases-and-conditions/glycemic-index-and-glycemic-load-for-100-foods

23. American Heart Association, 2017. Dietary Fats and Cardiovascular Disease A Presidential Advisory from the American Heart Association. Retrieved from: https://www.ahajournals.org/doi/pdf/10.1161/CIR.0000000000000510

24. Simopoulos, 2006. Evolutionary aspects of diet, the omega-6/omega-3 ratio and genetic variation: nutritional implications for chronic diseases. Retrieved from: https://pubmed.ncbi.nlm.nih.gov/17045449/

25. Patterson et al 2012. Health Implications of High Dietary Omega-6 Polyunsaturated Fatty Acids. Retrieved from: https://www.ncbi.nlm.nih.gov/pmc/articles/PMC3335257/

26. Lorgeril et al. 1999. Mediterranean diet, traditional risk factors, and the rate of cardiovascular complications after myocardial infarction: final report of the Lyon Diet Heart Study retrieved from: https://www.ncbi.nlm.nih.gov/pubmed/9989963?dopt=Abstract

27. Estruch et al. 2013. 'Primary Prevention of Cardiovascular Disease with a Mediterranean Diet'. Retrieved from: https://www.nejm.org/doi/full/10.1056/nejmoa1200303

28. Ibarrola-Jurado et al 2013. Cross-Sectional Assessment of Nut Consumption and Obesity, Metabolic Syndrome and Other Cardiometabolic Risk Factors: The PREDIMED Study. Retrieved from: https://www.ncbi.nlm.nih.gov/pmc/articles/PMC3583833/

29. Storniolo CE[1] et al. 2015. A Mediterranean diet supplemented with extra virgin olive oil or nuts improves endothelial markers involved in blood pressure control in hypertensive women. https://europepmc.org/article/med/26450601

30. Casas et al, 2014. The Effects of the Mediterranean Diet on Biomarkers of Vascular Wall Inflammation and Plaque Vulnerability in Subjects with High Risk for Cardiovascular Disease. A Randomized Trial. Retrieved from: https://www.ncbi.nlm.nih.gov/pmc/articles/PMC4055759/

31. Mark Hyman, 2016. 'Eat Fat Get Thin: Why the Fat We Eat Is the Key to Sustained Weight Loss and Vibrant Health'. Yellow Kite (29 Dec. 2016).

32. Czeglédi E, 2016. '[Options for stress management in obesity treatment]' Retrieved from: https://www.ncbi.nlm.nih.gov/pubmed/26853727

33. Raspopow, et al. 2013. 'Unsupportive social interactions influence emotional eating behaviors. The role of coping styles as mediators'. Retrieved from: https://pubmed.ncbi.nlm.nih.gov/23228905/

34. Young and Limbers, 2017. Avoidant coping moderates the relationship between stress and depressive emotional eating in adolescents. Retrieved from: https://www.ncbi.nlm.nih.gov/pubmed/28493151

35. Kanherkar et al 2017. Epigenetic Mechanisms of Integrative Medicine. Retrieved from: https://www.ncbi.nlm.nih.gov/pmc/articles/PMC5339524/

36. Acharya Balkrishna, 2015. A Practical Approach to the Science of Ayurveda: A Comprehensive Guide for Healthy Living. Lotus Press; Illustrated edition (16 Sept. 2015).

Joyful Movement

1. Kavanagh T, et al.2002. 'Prediction of Long-Term Prognosis in 12169 Men Referred for Cardiac Rehabilitation. Retrieved from: https://pubmed.ncbi.nlm.nih.gov/12163425/

2. Association of Chartered Physiotherapists in Cardiac Rehabilitation. Standards for Physical Activity and Exercise in the Cardiovascular Population, 2015. Retrieved from: https://www.acpicr.com/data/Page_Downloads/ACPICRStandards.pdf

3. Taylor RS, et al. 2004. Exercise-based rehabilitation for people with coronary heart disease: systematic review and meta-analysis of randomized controlled trials. Retrieved from: https://pubmed.ncbi.nlm.nih.gov/15121495/

4. Blaha et al, 2015. Age-dependent prognostic value of exercise capacity and derivation of fitness-associated biologic age. Retrieved from: https://heart.bmj.com/content/heartjnl/102/6/431.full.pdf

5. Schmid et al. 2018. 'Yoga improves quality of life and fall-risk factors in a sample of people with chronic pain and type 2 diabetes'. Retrieved from: https://www.sciencedirect.com/science/article/abs/pii/S1744388117304383

6. Yoshihara et al. 2014. Effect of 12 weeks of yoga training on the somatization, psychological symptoms, and stress-related biomarkers of healthy women. Retrieved from: https://pubmed.ncbi.nlm.nih.gov/23930028/

7. Sengupta, 2012. 'Health Impacts of Yoga and Pranayama: A State-of-the-Art Review. Retrieved from: https://www.ncbi.nlm.nih.gov/pmc/articles/PMC3415184/ 10.

Chapter 8: Sleep

1. Morgenthaler et al. 2015. 'Development of the National Healthy Sleep Awareness Project: Sleep Health Surveillance Questions. Retrieved from: https://www.researchgate.net/publication/280630167_Development_ of_the_National_Healthy_Sleep_Awareness_Project_Sleep_Health_S urveillance_Questions

2. Colten, and Altevogt, 2006. 'Sleep Disorders and Sleep Deprivation: An Unmet Public Health Problem' Retrieved from: https://pubmed.ncbi.nlm.nih.gov/20669438/

3. Xiao et al. 2013. A Large Prospective Investigation of Sleep Duration, Weight Change, and Obesity in the NIH-AARP Diet and Health Study Cohort. Retrieved from: https://academic.oup.com/aje/article/178/11/1600/83147

4. Patel et al. 2006. 'Association between Reduced Sleep and Weight Gain in Women'. Retrieved from: https://www.ncbi.nlm.nih.gov/pmc/articles/PMC3496783/

5. Harvard Health Publishing. A good night's sleep: Advice to take to heart: irregular or insufficient sleep increases your risk of cardiovascular disease. Retrieved from: https://www.health.harvard.edu/heart-health/a-good-nights-sleep-advice-to-take-to-heart

6. GRANDNER, et al. 2013. 'Sleep disturbance is associated with cardiovascular and metabolic disorders'. Retrieved from: https://www.ncbi.nlm.nih.gov/pmc/articles/PMC3703752/

7. GRANDNER, et al. 2016. 'Sleep: important considerations for the prevention of cardiovascular disease'. Retrieved from: https://www.ncbi.nlm.nih.gov/pubmed/27467177

8. Foster et al. 2009. 'Obstructive Sleep Apnea Among Obese Patients With Type 2 Diabetes'. Retrieved from:

https://care.diabetesjournals.org/content/32/6/1017.abstract

9. Alvaro et al, 2017. 'The direction of the relationship between symptoms of insomnia and psychiatric disorders in adolescents'. Retrieved from: https://www.researchgate.net/publication/308944836_The_direction _of_the_relationship_between_symptoms_of_insomnia_and_psychi atric_disorders_in_adolescents

10. Harvey et al. 2009. 'Sleep Disturbance in Bipolar Disorder Across the Lifespan.' Retrieved from: https://www.ncbi.nlm.nih.gov/pmc/articles/PMC3321357/

Section 3:

1. BJ Fogg, 2019. 'Tiny Habits: The Small Changes That Change Everything'. Virgin Books (31 Dec. 2019).

2. Eckhart Tolle, 2020. 'The Power of Now: A Guide to Spiritual Enlightenment'. Yellow Kite; 1st edition (9 Jan. 2020)

3. Oppong 2017. 'This is How to Increase The Odds of Reaching Your Goals by 95%'. Retrieved from: https://medium.com/the-mission/the-accountability-effect-a-simple-way-to-achieve-your-goals-and-boost-your-performance-8a07c76ef53a

4. STEEL, P, 2011. 'The Nature of Procrastination – A Meta-Analytic and Theoretical Review of Quintessential Self-Regulatory Failure'. Retrieved from: https://www.scribd.com/doc/63679278/STEEL-P-The-Nature-of-Procrastination-A-Meta- Analytic-and-Theoretical-Review-of-Quintessential-Self-Regulatory-Failure

Section 4

1. Rainforth et al, 2007. 'Stress reduction programs in patients with elevated blood pressure: a systematic review and meta-analysis'. Retrieved from: https://www.ncbi.nlm.nih.gov/pubmed/18350109?dopt=Abstract

2. Levine,et al. 2017. 'Meditation and Cardiovascular Risk Reduction: A Scientific Statement from the American Heart Association'. Retrieved from: https://www.ahajournals.org/doi/full/10.1161/JAHA.117.002218

3. Kemeny et al, 2011. 'Contemplative/emotion training reduces negative emotional behavior and promotes prosocial responses'. Retrieved from: https://pubmed.ncbi.nlm.nih.gov/22148989/

4. Manocha et al, 2011. 'A Randomized, Controlled Trial of Meditation for Work Stress, Anxiety and Depressed Mood in Full-Time Workers'. Retrieved from: https://www.hindawi.com/journals/ecam/2011/960583/

5. Hölzel et al, 2011. 'Mindfulness practice leads to increases in regional brain gray matter density'. Retrieved from: https://www.sciencedirect.com/science/article/abs/pii/S09254927100 0288X

6. Dan Buettner, 2008. 'The Blue Zones: Lessons for Living Longer From the People Who've Lived the Longest.' National Geographic; 1st edition (March 25, 2008).

7. Wu et al. 2016. 'The Association of Retirement Age with Mortality: A Population-Based Longitudinal Study among Older Adults in the United States'. Retrieved from: https://www.ncbi.nlm.nih.gov/pmc/articles/PMC6524971/

8. Fitzpatrick and Moore, 2018. 'The Mortality Effects of Retirement: Evidence from Social Security Eligibility at Age 62' Retrieved from:

https://www.sciencedirect.com/science/article/abs/pii/S0047272717302037

9. https://bmccomplementmedtherapies.biomedcentral.com/articles/10.1186/s12906-0182275-9

Acknowledgements

Thank you, dear readers, for sharing your time and enjoying this journey with me. Writing this book was one of the most important inspired actions I have taken; it has helped me grow as a person and a practitioner.

Thank you to many incredible people around the world who gave me the opportunity to play a small part in their healing journey and in turn allowed me to learn myriad aspects of human dynamics as it relates to healing and wellness.

Thank you to my dear mum in heaven, who worked hard to ensure my mind is growing and pursuing my wild dreams that can make a positive impact in the world. Thank you to my dad who is my constant source of unconditional love, who is there for me through the joys and tears of life with his warm smile and kind heart. I owe you both my everything.

Thank you for many teachers in my life who gave me the strength of knowledge and wisdom. Thank you to my high school teacher, Mrs Vaidya, who believed in my larger-than-life vision and my ability to achieve it. Mrs Vaidya, thank you for your blessings.

Thank you to Professor Wood, and other teachers of Imperial College London for their knowledge and wisdom, and for helping me regain my confidence in my skills to start my entrepreneurial journey in health and wellness.

I express my gratitude to my editor and publisher, Stephanie Hale, for her patience, positive feedback and encouragement through-out the process of completion of my book.

Thank you to everyone who has supported me throughout my journey.

Thank you, Divine Power for flowing through me when I am writing and when I am an instrument of transformation for those who need my help.

Love and gratitude,

Pranita

Author Biography

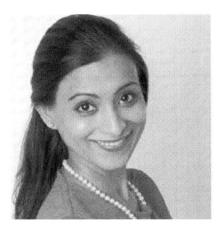

Pranita Salunke is the founder of Pranita Vitality – helping individuals to have a strong mind and a healthy heart that beats stronger for longer.

With two decades of clinical experience as an Occupational Therapist and Preventive Cardiology Specialist, including working for National Health Services, UK, Pranita has helped many people on both sides of healthcare – prevention and reactive.

Pranita is also the creator of the Vitality Mind-Body-Connection (MBC) approach, a unique combination of modern medicine (Occupational Therapy and Preventive Cardiology) and ancient well-being philosophies.

She is a lifelong learner of yoga, mindfulness and meditation, the practices that helped her personally to improve her well-being.

These principles have helped many people to lose up to 5 stones of weight, reverse type 2 diabetes and prediabetes, enhance energy, improve their cognitive skills, increase productivity, and made them feel youthful and happy.

Pranita strongly believes that great health is not only our birthright but also our number one responsibility.

Experiencing the personal loss of loved ones to uncontrolled diabetes, and after helping herself to overcome mental distress and its impact on her body, she strongly believes that **it's our lifestyle and mindset that sets us on the path miraculous healing.**

Pranita promotes this message by speaking across communities, including corporate organisations and the UK Parliament.

She has founded Pranita Vitality, a lifestyle transformation service, with the intention of helping humanity and fulfilling her vision: **"to reduce the global threat of chronic diseases by inspiring, educating and empowering people to transform their lifestyle.** As a result, they can enjoy life to the full, fulfil their purpose and leave the legacy for which they have been placed on this planet."

In her spare time, Pranita enjoys spending time with her son and family, and loves to travel to beautiful destinations. She also enjoys long nature walks, adventurous activities like water sports, and trekking. She also finds joy in the cultural pursuits of theatre, musicals and visiting many museums.

Her dream is to grow the Pranita Vitality movement so that it can support many charities, supporting children's well-being across the world – because, children are a gift to humanity and deserve love and nurturing to help them live to their fullest potential.

Next Steps

1. Visit https://pranitavitality.com/resources/ and download all the gifts that accompany this book, including your Self-assessment Questionnaire

2. Share your feedback by contacting me at: https://pranitavitality.com/contact-me/

3. Join me on Social Media:

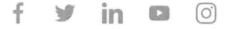

https://www.facebook.com/Pranitavitality

https://www.instagram.com/pranitavitality/

https://www.youtube.com/channel/UCscp38oQL6vpNQKGgC5ecQg?view_as=subscriber

https://www.linkedin.com/in/pranita-salunke-9a92873a/

https://twitter.com/Pranita211

4. Review this book on Amazon.

Importantly:
Live well – Live with Vitality!

Praise

"To be successful in business and life, you need to have a healthy body and happy mind. In this book, Pranita guides us to reach that destination. You deserve this book!"
—Daniel Priestley, author of four best-selling entrepreneurship books and co-founder of Dent Global, a leading business accelerator in the UK, Australia and Canada. He's named in the Top 10 Business Advisors in the UK.

"A life-changing practical book to help you lose weight and prevent type 2 diabetes with excellent lifestyle tools! Read this book to learn Pranita's practical and compassionate approach for optimum wellness."
—Dr Aseem Malhotra. Cardiologist, Sunday Times best-selling author, researcher and Professor of Evidence-Based Medicine.

"A labour of love from a determined and focused individual trying to make a change to people's lives! All the very best for this and future endeavours."
—Professor Parth Kar, National Specialty Advisor, Diabetes NHS England, Diabetes Lead NHS GIRFT and Consultant Endocrinologist, NHS.

"Transformational! I worked with Pranita for six months and during this period, my health has improved markedly, losing 18kg in weight, reversing pre-diabetes, and reducing a lot of arthritic pain that I had previously suffered from. Pranita's holistic approach means that all aspects of my life have been enriched beyond recognition. My mindset is the most powerful and focused that I can remember in over ten years. Thank you Pranita."
—Paul Tabron, Managing Partner PJT Accountancy

Printed in Great Britain
by Amazon